T0077834

Praise for *Cr*

"Watters commands attention with manner while drawing much-needed attention to the consequences of Western intrusion. This fascinating book deserves attention from mental health workers and Americans interested in the reach of their culture's psyche across the globe."

—*Library Journal*

"In the best investigative reporting tradition . . . Ethan Watters stirs up one controversy after another in this provocative study of mental illness diagnosis and treatment in cultures other than our own."

—*Shelf Awareness*

"In crisp journalistic style, Watters argues convincingly that what the American psychiatric industry exports is not so much drugs as diseases."

—*Mother Jones*

"I couldn't put it down. *Crazy Like Us* is a fascinating and provocative intellectual travelogue, and Watters is a fearless guide."

—**Alan Burdick, author of *Out of Eden***

"Ethan Watters has traveled the world to look at how globalization reaches far beyond economics, and into people's very conceptions of what constitutes health and sanity. I find his book provocative, original, and convincing."

—**Adam Hochschild, author of *Bury the Chains* and *King Leopold's Ghost***

"Searing, startling, and utterly unforgettable. Ethan Watters brilliantly surveys the stark interior cost of globalization, from our export of stress disorders to Sri Lanka to our marketing of depression in Japan as 'a cold of the soul.' *Crazy Like Us* is a grand tour of the new global psyche, distorted and darkened by the export of the American dream."

—**Jason Roberts, National Book Critics Circle finalist for *A Sense of the World***

"A devastating account of America's psychological adventures abroad. The stories Watters tells will move you, surprise you, and occasionally infuriate you, and they will change the way you think about culture, human nature, and the mind."

—**Paul Tough, author of *Whatever It Takes***

ALSO BY ETHAN WATTERS

Urban Tribes:
A Generation Redefines Friendship,
Family, and Commitment

WITH RICHARD OFSHE

Makings Monsters:
False Memories, Psychotherapy, and Sexual Hysteria

CRAZY LIKE US

THE GLOBALIZATION OF
THE AMERICAN PSYCHE

ETHAN WATTERS

FREE PRESS

New York London Toronto Sydney

*f*P

FREE PRESS

A Division of Simon & Schuster, Inc.
1230 Avenue of the Americas
New York, NY 10020

Copyright © 2010 by Ethan Watters

All rights reserved, including the right to reproduce this book or
portions thereof in any form whatsoever. For information address
Free Press Subsidiary Rights Department, 1230 Avenue of the Americas,
New York, NY 10020

First Free Press trade paperback edition March 2011

FREE PRESS and colophon are trademarks of Simon & Schuster, Inc.

For information about special discounts for bulk purchases,
please contact Simon & Schuster Special Sales at 1-866-506-1949 or
business@simonandschuster.com.

The Simon & Schuster Speakers Bureau can bring authors to your live event.
For more information or to book an event contact the Simon & Schuster
Speakers Bureau at 1-866-248-3049 or visit our website at
www.simonspeakers.com.

Manufactured in the United States of America

19   20

The Library of Congress has catalogued the hardcover edition as follows:
Watters, Ethan.
Crazy like us: the globalization of the American psyche / Ethan Watters.
p. cm.
1. Mental illness—Cross-cultural studies. 2. Psychology, Pathological—
Cross-cultural studies. 3. Irish—Race identity. 4. Mental illness—
United States. 5. Globalization—Psychological aspects. 6. Psychiatric
epidemiology. I. Title.
RC455.4.E8W38   2010
616.89—dc22   2009030661
ISBN 978-1-4165-8708-8
ISBN 978-1-4165-8709-5 (pbk)
ISBN 978-1-4165-8719-4 (ebook)

For my mother, Mary Pulliam Watters

Contents

CRAZY LIKE US

Introduction

To travel internationally is to become increasingly unnerved by the way American culture pervades the world. We cringe at the new indoor Mlimani shopping mall in Dar es Salaam, Tanzania. We shake our heads at the sight of a McDonald's on Tiananmen Square or a Nike factory in Malaysia. The visual landscape of the world has become depressingly familiar. For Americans the old joke has become bizarrely true: wherever we go, there we are.

We have the uneasy feeling that our influence over the rest of the world is coming at a great cost: loss of the world's diversity and complexity. For all our self-incrimination, however, we have yet to face our most disturbing effect on the rest of the world. Our golden arches do not represent our most troubling impact on other cultures; rather, it is how we are flattening the landscape of the human psyche itself. We are engaged in the grand project of Americanizing the world's understanding of the human mind.

This might seem like an impossible claim to back up, as such a change would be happening inside the conscious and unconscious thoughts of more than six billion people. But there are telltale signs that have recently become unmistakable. Particularly telling are the changing manifestations of mental illnesses around the world. In the past two decades, for instance, eating disorders have risen in Hong Kong and are now spreading to inland China. Post-traumatic

1

stress disorder (PTSD) has become the common diagnosis, the lingua franca of human suffering, following wars and natural disasters. In addition, a particularly Americanized version of depression is on the rise in countries across the world.

What is the pathogen that has led to these outbreaks and epidemics? On what currents do these illnesses travel?

The premise of this book is that the virus is us.

Over the past thirty years, we Americans have been industriously exporting our ideas about mental illness. Our definitions and treatments have become the international standards. Although this has often been done with the best of intentions, we've failed to foresee the full impact of these efforts. It turns out that how a people in a culture think about mental illnesses—how they categorize and prioritize the symptoms, attempt to heal them, and set expectations for their course and outcome—influences the diseases themselves. In teaching the rest of the world to think like us, we have been, for better and worse, homogenizing the way the world goes mad.

There is now a remarkable body of research that suggests that mental illnesses are not, as sometimes assumed, spread evenly around the globe. They have appeared in different cultures in endlessly complex and unique forms. Indonesian men have been known to experience *amok*, in which a minor social insult launches an extended period of brooding punctuated by an episode of murderous rage. Southeastern Asian males sometimes suffer from *koro*, the debilitating certainty that their genitals are retracting into their body. Across the Fertile Crescent of the Middle East there is *zar*, a mental illness related to spirit possession that brings forth dissociative episodes of crying, laughing, shouting, and singing.

The diversity that can be found across cultures can be seen across time as well. Because the troubled mind has been perceived in terms of diverse religious, scientific, and social beliefs of discrete cultures, the forms of madness from one place and time in history often look remarkably different from the forms of madness in another. These differing forms of mental illness can sometimes appear and disappear within a generation. In his book *Mad Travelers,* Ian Hacking documents the fleeting appearance in Victorian Europe of a fugue state in which young men would walk in a trance for hundreds of miles. Symptoms of mental illnesses are the lightning in the zeitgeist, the product of culture and belief in specific times and specific places. That thousands of upper-class women in the mid-nineteenth century couldn't get out of bed due to the onset of hysterical leg paralysis gives us a visceral understanding of the restrictions set on women's social roles at the time.

But with the increasing speed of globalization, something has changed. The remarkable diversity once seen among different cultures' conceptions of madness is rapidly disappearing. A few mental illnesses identified and popularized in the United States—depression, post-traumatic stress disorder, and anorexia among them—now appear to be spreading across cultural boundaries and around the world with the speed of contagious diseases. Indigenous forms of mental illness and healing are being bulldozed by disease categories and treatments made in the USA.

There is no doubt that the Western mental health profession has had a remarkable global influence over the meaning and treatment of mental illness. Mental health professionals trained in the West, and in the United States in particular, create the official categories of mental diseases. The American Psychiatric Association's *Diagnostic and Statistical Manual of Mental Disorders,* the *DSM* (the "bible" of the profession, as it is sometimes called), has become the worldwide standard. In addition American researchers and organizations run the premier scholarly journals and host top conferences in the fields of psychology and psychiatry. Western universities train the world's most influential clinicians and academics. Western drug companies dole out the funds for research and spend billions marketing medications for mental illnesses. Western-trained traumatologists rush in wherever war or natural disasters strike to deliver "psychological first aid," bringing with them their assumptions about how the mind becomes broken and how it is best healed.

These ideas and practices represent much more than the symptom lists that describe these conditions. Behind the promotion of Western ideas of mental health and healing lies a variety of cultural assumptions about human nature itself. Westerners share, for instance, beliefs about what type of life event is likely to make one psychologically traumatized, and we agree that venting emotions by talking is more healthy than stoic silence. We are certain that humans are innately fragile and should consider many emotional experiences as illnesses that require professional intervention. We're confident that our biomedical approach to mental illness will reduce stigma for the sufferer and that our drugs are the best that science has to offer. We promise people in other cultures that mental health (and a modern style of self-awareness) can be found by throwing off traditional social roles and engaging in individualistic quests of introspection. These Western ideas of the mind are proving as seductive to the rest of the world as fast food and rap music, and we are spreading them with speed and vigor.

What motivates us in this global effort to convince the world to think like us? There are several answers to this question, but one of them is quite simple: drug company profits. These multibillion-dollar conglomerates have an incentive to promote universal disease categories because they can make fortunes selling the drugs that purport to cure those illnesses.

Other reasons are more complex. Many modern mental health practitioners and researchers believe that the science behind our drugs, our illness categories, and our theories of the mind have put the field beyond the influence of constantly shifting cultural trends and beliefs. After all, we now have machines that can literally watch the mind at work. We can change the chemistry of the brain in a variety of ways and examine DNA sequences for abnormalities. For a generation now we have proudly promoted the biomedical notion of mental illness: the idea that these diseases should be understood clinically and scientifically, like physical illnesses. The assumption is that these remarkable scientific advances have allowed modern-day practitioners to avoid the biases and mistakes of their predecessors.

Indeed modern-day mental health practitioners often look back at previous generations of psychiatrists with a mixture of scorn and pity, wondering how they could have been so swept away by the cultural beliefs of their time. Theories surrounding the epidemic of hysterical women in the Victorian era are now dismissed as cultural artifacts. Even recent iatrogenic contagions, such as the sudden rise of multiple personality disorder just fifteen years ago, are considered ancient history, harmful detours but safely in the past. Similarly, illnesses found only in other cultures are often treated like carnival sideshows. *Koro* and *amok* and the like can be found far back in the American diagnostic manual (*DSM-IV*, pages 845–849) under the heading "Culture-Bound Syndromes." They might as well be labeled "Psychiatric Exotica: Two Bits a Gander."

Western mental health practitioners are prone to believe that, unlike those culturally contrived manifestations of mental illness, the 844 pages of the *DSM-IV* prior to the inclusion of culture-bound syndromes describe *real* disorders of the mind, illnesses with symptomatology and outcomes relatively unaffected by shifting cultural beliefs. And, the logic goes, if they are unaffected by culture, then these disorders are surely universal to humans everywhere. Their application around the world therefore represents simply the brave march of scientific knowledge.

But the cross-cultural researchers and anthropologists profiled in this book have a different story to tell. They have shown that the experience of mental illness cannot be separated from culture. We can become psychologically unhinged for many reasons, such as personal trauma, social upheaval, or a chemical imbalance in our brain. Whatever the cause, we invariably rely on cultural beliefs and stories to understand what is happening. Those stories, whether they tell of spirit possession or serotonin depletion, shape the experience of the illness in surprisingly dramatic and often counterintuitive ways. In the end, all mental illnesses, including such seemingly obvious categories such as depression, PTSD, and even schizophrenia, are every bit as shaped and influenced by cultural beliefs and expectations as hysterical leg paralysis, or the vapors, or *zar*, or any other mental illness ever experienced in the history of human madness.

The cultural influence on the mind of a mentally ill person is always a local and intimate phenomenon. So although this book describes a global trend, it is not told from a global perspective. In the hopes of keeping the human-scale impact in sight, I have chosen to tell the stories of four diseases in four different countries. I picked these tales because each illustrates how the globalization of Western beliefs about mental health travel on different currents. From the island of Zanzibar, where beliefs in spirit possession are increasingly giving way to biomedical notions of mental illness, I tell the story of two families struggling with schizophrenia. To document the rise of anorexia in Hong Kong, I retrace the last steps of 14-year-old Charlene Hsu Chi-Ying and show how the publicity surrounding her death introduced the province to a particularly Western form of the disease. I deconstruct the mega-marketing of the antidepressant Paxil in Japan to illustrate how drug companies often sell the very disease for which their drug purports to be a cure. The aftermath of the 2004 tsunami in Sri Lanka provides the opportunity to examine the impact of trauma counselors who rush into disaster zones armed with the diagnosis of posttraumatic stress and Western certainties about the impact of trauma on the human psyche.

At the end of each of these chapters I turn the focus back to the West, and to the United States in particular. When viewed from a far shore, the cultural assumptions and certainties that shape our own beliefs about mental illness and the human mind often become breathtakingly clear. From this perspective, it is often our own assumptions about madness and the self that begin to appear truly strange.

The cross-cultural psychiatrists and anthropologists featured in this book have convinced me that we are living at a remarkable moment in human history. At the same time they've been working hard to document the different cultural understandings of mental illness and health, those differences have been disappearing before their eyes. I've come to think of them as psychology's version of botanists in the rain forest, desperate to document the diversity while staying only a few steps ahead of the bulldozers.

We should worry about this loss of diversity in the world's differing conceptions and treatments of mental illness in exactly the same way we worry about the loss of biological diversity in nature. Modes of healing and culturally specific beliefs about how to achieve mental health can be lost to humanity with the grim finality of an animal or plant lapsing into extinction. And like those plants and animals, the diversity in the human understanding of the mind can disappear before we've truly comprehended its value. Biologists suggest that within the dense and vital biodiversity of the rain forest are chemical compounds that may someday cure modern plagues. Similarly, within the diversity of different cultural understandings of mental health and illness may exist knowledge that we cannot afford to lose. We erase this diversity at our own peril.

1

The Rise of Anorexia in Hong Kong

Psychiatric theory cannot deny its participation in the social trajectory of the anorectic discourse, which articulates personal miseries as much as it does public concerns.

SING LEE

On the morning of my visit to Dr. Sing Lee, China's preeminent researcher on eating disorders, I took the subway a few stops north of downtown Hong Kong to the Prince of Wales Hospital in the suburb of Shatin. In the clean and well-lit subway corridors, I passed several large posters featuring outlandishly slender, bikinied young women promoting a variety of health care regimens, cellulite-removing creams, and appetite-suppressant supplements. The advertisements over the handrails in the subway cars repeated the offers. The magazines and newspapers being read by the commuters were filled with similar pitches, often featuring before and after photos, young women becoming little more than skin and bones after the offered treatment. Such products are a huge business in Hong Kong and increasingly in mainland China. Over the past few years the beauty industry in Hong Kong (including dieting, cosmetics, skin care, and fitness) has outspent every other business sector on advertising. In that week's issue of the popular weekly magazine *Next*, a remarkable 110 of the publication's 150 ads were for slimming or beauty products and services.

The reporting and photojournalism that appeared alongside those ads had a slightly different obsession: telling tales of young women celebrities. That morning's *Standard*, one of Hong Kong's English dailies, prominently reported the recent misadventures of several famous young women, including Britney Spears, who had that week been held against her will at the UCLA Medical Center. She had been "5150ed," which is the code for a California statute that allows doctors to hold a patient involuntarily if she is deemed a danger to herself or others. On the opposing page was an article about the Japanese pop idol Kumi Koda, who lost her job as a spokesmodel for Japan's third largest cosmetics company, Kose Corp., after making pejorative comments about the fertility of older women. The cute and perky 25-year-old had gone on a popular radio show and given her medical opinion that a "mother's amniotic fluid turns rotten once a woman reaches about thirty-five . . . It gets dirty."

The biggest story in *The Standard*, in fact the front-page story in every paper in Hong Kong that morning, was a sex scandal involving a handful of the region's best-known female pop stars and a young actor. Hundreds of very explicit nude photos had been posted on the Internet of singer Gillian Chung and actresses Bobo Chen and Cecilia Cheung Pak-chi, among a dozen others. That same week a humanitarian crisis was erupting along the Gaza-Egyptian border and a severe snowstorm was sweeping across much of eastern China, threatening to strand millions of holiday travelers, yet no other story could compete with this sex scandal. Everyone, from politicians to op-ed writers, felt the need to criticize the behavior of the young women. Even Hong Kong's Catholic bishop John Tong weighed in on the subject of celebrity sin and cyber etiquette, saying that it was important to "keep our minds decent" and "not post or circulate these pictures."

Of course it's not possible to say exactly what these advertisements, images, and stories of celebrity misadventures might have been adding up to in the minds of average adolescent girls in Hong Kong. It didn't take much reading between the lines, however, to perceive a high degree of confusion and ambivalence surrounding the issues of female body image, sexuality, youth, beauty, and aging. Young women in some contexts were worshipped for their attractiveness, while in other situations they were humiliated and publicly vilified with a vitriol that would be hard to overstate. Whatever understanding Hong Kong teenage girls were piecing together about the postadolescent world from these sources, it is safe to say that it was not unconflicted.

Given this environment, it would make sense to most Americans and Europeans that occurrences of anorexia and bulimia have spiked here in the past fifteen years. Nor would it likely be a surprise that Gillian Chung, one of those young celebrities in the sex scandal, had herself battled bulimia. Most well-educated Westerners understand that anorexia is sparked by cultural cues, but they often have a fairly narrow conception of what those cues might be. Most assume that anorexia, with its attendant fear of fatness and body dysmorphic disorder, is born of a peculiar modern fixation with a slender, female body type, and that popular culture transmits this fetish to young women. As we've exported our obsessions with slender models—our Barbie dolls and our Kate Moss fashions—it makes sense to us that eating disorders have followed in their wake.

But although this commonsense cause and effect might be part of the story, Sing Lee's research shows that there have been other, more subtle, cross-cultural forces at work here. The full story of how anorexia spread from the American suburbs to Hong Kong is more complex and, in many ways, more troubling. It turns out that the West may indeed be culpable for the rise in eating disorders in Asia, but not for the obvious reasons.

After making my way across Shatin, I found Lee's small suite of offices among the labyrinth of midrise buildings that make up the Prince of Wales Hospital. Introduced by his assistant, Dr. Lee was younger than I expected. At 49 years old, he's had a remarkable output as a scholar despite the fact that he has split his time between seeing patients at the public hospital, teaching, and running a mood disorders center. He admits that at times he has been accused of being a workaholic. "I do work long hours, but I've never experienced much work stress," he said to me in what I would come to know as his characteristic humble manner. "I've wanted to be a psychiatrist since high school and I still love the work of meeting patients and writing about ideas." Given the amount of time he spends in his office, he's allowed himself to build a comfortable environment. The place has the feel of a stylish bachelor pad. The bucket seat and gearshift of a sports car sat on the floor next to the couch. Directly across from his desk was one of his prized possessions: an antique vacuum tube stereo connected to two imposingly large speakers. The tuner was made in the early 1960s and at the time cost as much as a VW Beetle and requires vacuum tubes the size of small lightbulbs to operate. For a true classical music audiophile such as Lee, however, there is no substitute for the resonant tones it produces.

Even after two decades of charting the cultural currents that have brought the American version of anorexia to these shores, Lee remains passionately interested in talking about the puzzle. He was the first scholar to document anorexia in Chinese women. The remarkable thing he found was that before the illness was well known in the province, Chinese anorexia was unlike that found in the West. These atypical anorexics, as he calls them, displayed a different cluster of symptoms than their Western counterparts. Most, for instance, did not display the classic fear of fatness common among Western anorexics, nor did they misperceive the frail state of their body by believing they were overweight. It was while he was trying to puzzle out these differences that he witnessed something remarkable.

Over a short period of time the presentation of anorexia in Hong Kong changed. The symptom cluster that was unique to his Hong Kong patients began to disappear. What was once a rare disorder was replaced by an American version of the disease that became much more widespread. Understanding the forces behind that change may not only explain why anorexia became common in Hong Kong, but it may also lead us to reconsider the momentum behind the disease in the West.

The Death of a Patient

When Sing Lee came back to Hong Kong from his training in England in the mid-1980s, he took a job at the Prince of Wales Hospital and began looking for Chinese anorexics. Having been introduced to the disorder while in England he was, like many young psychiatrists, fascinated by the fundamental conundrum of the disease: Why would healthy young women with plenty of resources starve themselves?

At the time Lee began his search, the long-held belief that eating disorders were confined to American and Western European populations was just beginning to show cracks. Even though prominent eating disorder researchers were making the argument as late as 1985 that anorexia didn't exist outside of the United States, cases were beginning to show up in Russia and Eastern Europe. Although it was still believed to be rare in Latin American countries, researchers and clinicians also began discovering young women with anorexia in Japan and South Korea.

In China and Hong Kong the disorder remained all but unknown. Searching the two major psychiatric journals published in China, Lee found not a single paper documenting a Chinese woman with anorexia. With little to go on, he got to work searching the databases at the Prince of Wales Hospital. After an exhaustive search, he managed to identify just ten possible cases in the five years from 1983 to 1988. Given the thousands of patients seen at the hospital, he determined that anorexia was an exceedingly rare disorder in Hong Kong. His first paper on the topic, published in 1989 in the *British Journal of Psychiatry*, was titled "Anorexia Nervosa in Hong Kong: Why Not More in Chinese?"

The low rate of anorexia was a mystery that Lee wanted to figure out. Perhaps Chinese cultural beliefs or practices contained protective mechanisms. He knew, for instance, that historically there was little Chinese stigma surrounding larger body shapes. In fact popular Chinese sayings suggested that "being able to eat is to have luck," "gaining weight means good fortune," and "fat people have more luck." He also considered that the later onset of puberty in Chinese girls compared to girls in the West might be a preventive factor. The physical changes that come with puberty might be less psychologically stressful when experienced with an added year or two of emotional maturity.

But even taking these differences into account, Lee couldn't quite understand why the behavior was so uncommon among local adolescents. In many ways Hong Kong seemed primed for the disorder. It was a modern region that, thanks to years of British rule, had incorporated many Western values as well as styles of dress and eating. There were fast-food restaurants and health clubs. Thin Western and Chinese celebrities were idolized. It was a patriarchal culture, in which parents and teachers put intense pressure on students to compete. The Chinese obsession with food and the layered meanings of sharing meals within a family should have made food refusal a dangerously attractive behavior for an adolescent looking to send a distress signal to those around her.

All the triggers for anorexia that had been identified in Western literature seemed to be present in full force, and yet eating disorders remained rare. Lee suspected that there was something else, some factor that hadn't been fully considered in the Western literature, that remained absent in Hong Kong. What that factor might be he could only guess.

Treating the few cases he could find, Lee discovered another puzzle. He noticed that the women who starved themselves in Hong Kong were different from the anorexics he had studied while training in England. The variations were sometimes so pronounced he wondered if he was seeing the same disease. To illustrate those differences, Lee recounted to me the story of one of the first patients he personally treated, a 31-year-old saleswoman I'll call Jiao.

Lee still clearly remembers the first time he met Jiao in a hospital examination room in 1988. Although he knew from his research how thin anorexic patients could become, he couldn't help but be taken aback at the sight of her. "She was shockingly emaciated—virtually a skeleton," he recalls. "She had sunken eyes, hollow cheeks and pale, cold skin." She was alert but uncommunicative. At 5 feet 3 inches, her ideal body weight should have been in the neighborhood of 110 pounds. Indeed, she had been that weight four years earlier, before she began to waste away. By the time she sought medical treatment she weighed just 48 pounds.

During his physical exam of Jiao, Lee noted that she had dry skin and a subnormal body temperature. More concerning, her blood pressure was low and her heartbeat was a plodding 60 beats per minute. He took X-rays after giving her a drink laced with barium so he could examine her esophagus. He also used an endoscope to examine her upper gastrointestinal system for blockages or lesions. Convinced the disorder wasn't organic in origin, he began to piece together her personal history.

Jiao was the youngest child of three living children (two of her brothers died soon after birth). She had grown up in a working-class family in a rural village near Hong Kong, where she still lived. Like many in the Hong Kong area, her family was both emotionally enmeshed and yet physically disjointed. To earn a living, her father had lived apart from the family for many years at a time, but when he was present, he demanded the absolute loyalty he felt was his traditional due as head of the household. During his visits home he often berated Jiao and her mother for small infractions, such as interrupting him when he spoke, and he freely expressed his disappointment that Jiao had not performed better in school. Her mother was a traditional housewife who was subservient to her husband and was socially isolated because she spoke only a Chinese dialect called Hakka. Although it was not a happy home, there was no history of mental illness, sexual or physical abuse, or eating disorders.

Jiao's struggles with eating had begun in earnest four years earlier, in 1984, when her boyfriend deserted her by emigrating to England. She was devastated by his departure and began to refuse food and skip meals. Explaining her change in eating patterns to her family, she complained of pain and discomfort in her abdomen. During this time she became increasingly socially withdrawn and lost her job. Over those first years of the illness she saw various doctors. She was encouraged by health professionals as well as her family to eat more. Nevertheless she steadily lost weight year after year.

While relating her personal history to Lee during that first interview, Jiao cried at times but for the most part just looked sad and tired.

"What do you think is your main problem?" Lee finally asked her.

"Abdominal fullness and thinness," she replied.

"What else?"

"A bad mood, it's hard to describe. . . . It is no use talking about it anymore," she said and began to weep.

"Is there a name for your condition?" Lee asked her.

"I don't know," she said. "Can you tell me what kind of disease it is?"

Lee had her draw a picture of herself. This technique is often used to assess whether anorexic patients have a distorted perception of their emaciated condition. The stick figure sketch she handed back to Lee, however, closely matched her skeletal condition.

Jiao's presentation left Lee in a quandary. On the one hand, she was clearly starving herself to the point of death. On the other hand, she didn't fit many of the American diagnostic criteria for anorexia. The *Diagnostic and Statistical Manual of Mental Disorders,* published by the American Psychiatric Association—the third edition released in the late 1980s had quickly become the worldwide standard—stated that someone suffering from anorexia not only rigidly maintains an abnormally low body weight but expresses an "intense fear of becoming obese, even when underweight," and has a disturbed self-image, such as claiming to "feel fat when emaciated."

But Jiao did not express a fear of being overweight. In addition, she didn't have any misperception about the emaciated condition of her body. She described herself pretty much exactly as Lee saw her: as a very sick and dangerously thin young woman.

When he gave her the standard eating disorder questionnaire of the time, it also showed clear differences from what one would expect of an anorexic in the West. For instance, Jiao insisted that she never consciously restricted the amount of food she ate. Western anorexics, he knew, usually admitted to obsessing over food portions and quantities. When asked why she often went for whole days without eating, Jiao would say only that she felt no hunger and, pointing to the left side of her abdomen, describe how her stomach often felt distended.

These deviations from the Western diagnosis weren't unique to Jiao. Most of the Hong Kong anorexics Lee was able to interview or treat around this time similarly denied any fear of being fat or of intending to lose weight to become more attractive. They often spoke of their desire to get back to a normal body weight. When explaining their refusal to eat, they most often ascribed the behavior to physical causes such as bloating, blockages in their throat or digestion, or the feeling of fullness in their stomach and abdomen. Their often repeated claim that they had no appetite also ran counter to conceptions of the disease put forward by Western experts. Psychiatrist Hilde Bruch, who wrote one of the seminal books on anorexia, *The Golden Cage*, asserted that "patients with anorexia nervosa do not suffer from loss of appetite; on the contrary, they are frantically preoccupied with food and eating. In this sense they resemble other starving people."

As a group, these Hong Kong anorexics were different from their American counterparts in other ways as well. These were not the "golden girls" described in Western literature on eating disorders. Anorexia in the West was known to afflict well-to-do, popular, and promising young women who were sometimes perfectionists in other parts of their lives, such as school or sports. But Lee's patients were often from poor families and among the lower achievers in their schools. They also did not give any hint of the moral superiority sometimes observed in Western anorexics.

Most curiously, they were often from outlying villages, not a population that Lee suspected would be most influenced by the globalization of Western pop culture. They had not begun their self-starvation after reading diet books or engaging in the exercise fads of the day. His atypical anorexics were not among the young women in Hong Kong adopting *Flashdance* fashions or going to Jazzercise classes. If Western pop cultural influences were at the heart of this disorder, there were certainly populations in Hong Kong who should have been harder hit. Hong Kong was, and remains, the most international of cities, and there were plenty of groups of adolescents and young women fully engaging in Western fashion and pop culture. But Lee's patients did not come from these jet-setting subcultures.

While Lee had great respect for the clinical knowledge he had gained during his training in the West, he knew it posed a challenge as well. With the *DSM* becoming the world's diagnostic manual for mental illness, it was easy to gloss over different disease presentations to make them fit the Western standard. But Lee was convinced that the distinctions between the American presentation of anorexia and what he was witnessing in Hong Kong was a meaningful difference that could lead to new insights into the disorder. He knew that if he was going to understand what was happening with his Hong Kong patients, he was going to have to get to the bottom of those differences.

Yin, Yang, and Qi

Despite Lee's uncertainty about the diagnosis of anorexia, Jiao was clearly in need of immediate attention. With Lee's encouragement she checked into the hospital, but she proved to be a difficult patient. She used a shifting series of excuses to refuse the food offered by the dietitian. Lee speculated that her resistance to his ministrations might be bound up in the culture clash between Western and Chinese medicine. Hoping to hit a resonant cultural note that would lessen her resistance, he called in a Chinese herbalist and then a qigong master to participate in her treatment. The herbalist reported to Lee that Jiao's condition involved a variety of imbalances between the liver, the spleen, and the stomach. Her extreme sadness over her lost love had caused her liver function to break down, the herbalist explained, which in turn had thrown off the workings of her spleen and stomach. This had resulted in poor absorption of food nutrition, limiting her body's ability to transform food into *qi,* the flow of energy that animates all living things. These problems had led to a weak heart and ineffective kidneys. In addition, the herbalist found a general imbalance in her system that he described as an excess of *yin* and a depleted reserve of *yang.*

Because the liver malfunction was at the beginning of the cascade of internal distress, the herbalist recommended a mixture of herbs he said would selectively soothe and repair that organ. The treatment, Jiao was told, would allow her to let go of the unhealthy energy that surrounded the memory of her lost love. Jiao refused to drink the concoction.

The qigong master was even less successful. He also believed that Jiao's flow of qi was dangerously low. He performed rituals to unblock her pent-up qi. By the third treatment, the qigong master quit the case, telling Lee that the patient was "not willing to recover."

With neither Western nor Eastern healing modalities having much impact, Jiao decided to leave the hospital. She was discharged just before Christmas of 1988. Although she had gained weight during her hospital stay, from 48 pounds to 59 pounds, in a checkup two weeks later she had already dropped four of those pounds. She refused readmission to the hospital and began to avoid outpatient visits as well. Over the next few years Lee twice visited her at home, hoping to lure her back into treatment. During this time her weight dropped back down to 50 pounds.

In 1992 Lee once again visited Jiao at home, taking two female medical students with him. Jiao looked as skeletal as ever and told of heart palpitations and lower limb weakness. Two of her front teeth had decayed to the point that they had been removed. Jiao's mother gestured to Lee that she was still not eating much. Because of the mother's language barrier, a neighbor was brought in to explain the need for inpatient treatment to her. The neighbor said that many in the village had tried unsuccessfully to encourage Jiao to eat more. The neighbor wanted to know from Lee what this mysterious disease was called and what caused it.

After the visit Lee and the two medical students took Jiao for a short walk in the village. She showed the students a picture of herself before the onset of the illness and seemed happy when they said she was pretty in the photos. She asked the students if they would reject her as a friend because of her current terrible appearance. At the end of the visit, Jiao agreed to consider returning to the hospital, but when Lee phoned her a few days later she declined again.

It was only two weeks later that Jiao showed up in the emergency room of the Prince of Wales Hospital. She was in terrible shape. She weighted only 42 pounds, her blood pressure was low, and sacral bedsores were appearing on her skin. She gasped for breath at the slightest exertion. To Lee's relief, Jiao agreed to hospitalization.

During her first day in the hospital, Lee noticed a positive turn in her outlook. Jiao asked for a referral to the occupational therapy department so that she could learn typing and computer skills. She hoped this would put her in line for a better job later in life. Some of the medical students who had been following her case with Dr. Lee gave her a present of a hat and scarf. The gift pleased Jiao. She asked to get a haircut and began to talk of "making a new beginning." She began to take small amounts of food orally.

Two days later, at four in the morning, Jiao's heart gave out. The autopsy showed no specific pathology other than multiple organ atrophy due to her self-starvation.

His failure to help Jiao recover fueled Lee's passion to figure out the meaning of anorexia in Hong Kong. Thinking back on the case, he became convinced that the Western understanding of the disease, focusing on body image and fat phobia, was of little use in cases like Jiao's. What was needed was not a global template for anorexia, but a much more local understanding of the personal and cultural forces at play. Relying on a global template, he believed, could be worse than just ineffective. The increasingly wide use of the Western diagnostic categories and the many assumptions that lay behind them had the potential of blinding local clinicians to the unique realities of patients in different cultures.

A Personal Test and Global Spread

Lee knew that he had to understand anorexia on two different levels. There was the question of why women began the behavior of self-starvation, and then there was the question of what happened to their mind and body as the regimen of starvation gained momentum in their daily life. Lee felt it was critically important to understand what anorexia felt like on a physiological level. "I was curious about the basic question: How can they eat so little?" Lee recalls. "Why did lunchtime make no difference to them? What did it mean to turn off the biological clock that signaled the body to eat?"

Empathy is prized among all mental health providers, but it's an ephemeral and untestable quality. A doctor may think he or she is sensing the internal world of the patient, but how can one really know? This is especially problematic when facing a patient with a severe mental illness. Can a doctor who treats a schizophrenic empathically connect with the workings of that patient's mind? Lee realized that, unlike in other mental disorders, a doctor treating an anorexic patient had some opportunity to share in the patient's experience. Because the key symptom—restricting one's eating—was an external behavior, Lee saw an opening to do an experiment. He decided to mimic the behavior of an anorexic in the early stages of the disorder.

"I got it in my head," says Lee, "that if I wanted to truly be an expert on this condition, I needed to experience it for myself." So he began to severely cut back on his food intake and skip lunch entirely. He also began an intense exercise routine. Like all dieters, at first he felt the normal drop in energy and mood as his body struggled to make it through the day with a depleted supply of calories. After a few weeks he had lost five pounds, but he still felt like he was dragging himself through his daily routine. After a month and a half of restricting food, he was another five pounds lighter but felt no better. His stomach ached and growled for food.

It was around the three-month mark that some gear shifted in his physiology. His energy began to return and his mood improved—more than improved, actually: he felt great. He was going to bed later and waking up earlier. He performed behaviors that he would have identified in a patient as potentially pathological. As he rode the elevator up to his office every morning, for instance, he did arm exercises on the handrails. He began to feel a hyperalertness and sense of mastery over his body and his life. For much of the day he was on the sort of pleasant runner's high that one feels in the middle of a good workout. His hunger, which for months had been sounding a deafening alarm, had become a background whisper that he could easily ignore.

He found himself feeling somewhat superior to other people, who seemed to be ruled by their incessant need for food. He couldn't understand why so many people who tried to diet lacked the willpower to do so. He found that he was inordinately pleased that he had the strength of will to see his project through. The next ten pounds came off with little effort and his friends and family began to comment on how thin he was. He had lost over 12 percent of his body weight.

Although Lee felt the desire to stay on his restrictive diet, he managed to shake himself out of the behavior. His excuse to himself at the time was that he needed to go to London for an intense exam at the Royal College of Psychiatry, and he worried that his lack of nutrition would limit his mental abilities. It had been a dangerous experiment but a successful one; he had heard a bit of the siren song that patients with anorexia often follow to their death.

One of his patients once told him that anorexia felt like getting on a train, only to discover too late that she was headed in the wrong direction. This patient felt she had little choice but to stay on that train to the final destination. Lee now had some idea what she meant when she used that metaphor to describe the psychological momentum that can build behind anorexia. He had starved himself to the point where the behavior can turn from a willful choice into a dangerous addiction.

As Lee's first papers on anorexia in Hong Kong moved toward publication, much was changing in the world of eating disorder research. Scattered case reports had been followed by outbreaks of eating disorders reported in Africa, India, and the Middle East. One study showed that students in Nigeria were scoring as high as Westerners on disordered eating scales. In the East, anorexia had become increasingly common in Taiwan, Malaysia, Singapore, and Japan.

The popular explanation at the time was that Western media were influencing the way women around the world viewed their bodies; as Western movie stars and models became the world standard for glamour and attractiveness, it appeared that eating disorders followed. Although that seemed like common sense, researchers who tried to prove a connection between Western acculturation and eating disorders were often frustrated. Usually these studies involved giving a group of immigrant women a test to measure abnormal eating attitudes, along with a set of questions intended to gauge their level of acculturation to their new home. The assumption was that women who had adopted Western norms would have higher scores on the disordered eating tests.

For the most part, however, these studies failed to make this seemingly commonsense cause-and-effect connection. In a review of eighteen such studies, a team of American researchers concluded, "Despite the long-standing hypothesis that a greater exposure to Western values leads to an increased risk for eating disorders, this review of acculturation research presents no compelling evidence for such a relationship." These researchers noted that the majority of studies failed to find a connection, and the few that did were offset by studies showing that immigrant women who were assimilated into Western culture sometimes had *lower* scores on disordered eating scales than women who held to their traditional beliefs and habits.

These latter studies that showed an inverse relationship between acculturation and disordered eating were the most controversial because they directly challenged the accepted wisdom that the true pathogen for eating disorders hid within Western attitudes toward the female body. Regardless, studies of British schoolgirls from South Asia consistently showed that those with a lower level of Western acculturation had *higher* levels of body dissatisfaction and eating disordered behavior. Strikingly similar results were found among Hong Kong–born women who moved to Australia.

It was clear that the pathogens that were spreading eating disorders around the world were not as simple as exposure to Western fashion, diets, or popular culture. What exactly was motivating the spread of the disorder remained a hot topic of debate. If, as Lee had discovered, local forms of anorexia were often markedly different from the *DSM* version of the disease, perhaps there weren't any universal causes for anorexia because it wasn't a single, unified disease. Or perhaps there was another spark for the spread of the disease that hadn't yet been considered.

The Mirror of History

Lee realized that his handful of Hong Kong patients represented a unique opportunity to examine an expression of anorexia divorced from Western cultural beliefs about the condition. Whereas it was all but impossible for a woman with an eating disorder in the United States to remain unaware of the various cultural meanings behind the behavior, Lee's Hong Kong atypicals often knew of no other sufferers and lacked even a name for their condition. They had come to the disease on their own and were negotiating a private meaning for their refusal to eat.

Hoping to glimpse the disease from a new perspective, Lee dove into the early history of the disorder. He became particularly interested in the work of a Canadian scholar named Edward Shorter, a medical historian who had recently written several influential papers on the history of anorexia. Reading the description of young women who starved themselves in the early to mid-nineteenth century, long before there was an official category for the illness, Lee was taken aback. The descriptions of those early self-starvers from more than a hundred years ago and half a world away sounded remarkably similar to the Hong Kong patients he was seeing in his practice.

Shorter recounts the story of a 16-year-old girl treated in 1823 by a Frankfurt physician named Salomon Stiebel. In Stiebel's account, the girl's troubles started when her parents insisted she break off a budding romantic relationship with a suitor they deemed inappropriate. After the girl was given the bad news "she felt a heavy pressure on the lower region of her esophagus, became pale and breathless, was unable to speak, and had to sit down." This feeling of pressure on her esophagus returned daily, making it impossible, she reported, for her to eat solid food. Although it seems clear that her self-starvation was psychological in origin—beginning as it did with the termination of a romance—the girl experienced her refusal to eat as a physical symptom: a literal blockage in her throat.

In his research Shorter reported a number of similar descriptions. Like Lee's patients in Hong Kong, these early anorexics reported a range of somatic reasons for refusing to eat. Echoing the explanations from Lee's patients, several nineteenth-century doctors reported that patients ascribed their food refusal to painful digestion. Many, like the girl in Frankfurt, told of the sensation of having an impassable lump in the throat. Food would "not go down," they would claim. Others claimed other physiological problems, such as the inability to chew.

These cases were interesting to Lee for what was absent. Like his atypical patients in Hong Kong, these early anorexics did not report a desire to lose weight, nor was there evidence that they had a fear of becoming fat. In addition these patients did not have a distorted body image, such as believing they were fat even though they were emaciated. Lee began to wonder whether he was seeing in his Hong Kong patients a rare pre-twentieth-century form of anorexia.

Shorter argued in his papers that the only way to understand the Western evolution of anorexia is to see it in the context of the archetypical psychological diagnosis of the nineteenth century: hysteria. Along with starving themselves, early anorexics often presented a number of classic symptoms of hysteria. This was true of the love-lorn girl from Frankfurt; her other symptoms of distress included pain at the slightest pressure on her sternum, numbness in one hand, and a persistent cough. She developed a facial tic and skin sensitivity on her face. She also experienced periods of catalepsy, a zombie-like state in which she heard what was going on around her but could not move or respond. Although this cluster of symptoms would look strange today, it would have been nothing new to the doctors of her time.

The middle decades of that century were a golden age for hysteria. At its high-water mark, hysteria could include a remarkable variety of symptoms: convulsive fits, paralysis, muscle contractions, linguistic impediments, amnesia, spinal irritation, day blindness, cold sensitivity, hallucinations, and astasia-abasia, the inability to stand or walk. The latest theories about the disease were often topics of conversations in upper-middle-class drawing rooms, where the latest editions of the *New England Journal of Medicine* and the *Lancet* could often be found. Like the Dr. Phils and Dr. Drews of our time, many practitioners in the Victorian era had a taste for the status and celebrity their positions offered them. Physicians such as Charles Laségue and Jean-Martin Charcot made their names by discovering in their patients novel manifestations of what was then the quintessential illness of womanhood. These doctors filled lecture halls to announce their discoveries and were toasted by royalty.

Documenting the rise of the disorder, historians such as Janet Oppenheim have given us a glimpse of how deeply hysteria influenced Victorian culture. Oppenheim found the disease not only in the mental health and medical literature of the time, but everywhere she looked. Popular magazines and newspapers, public hygiene literature, novels, short stories, personal letters, diaries, and autobiographies—it was an idea that had a tremendous hold on the population at the end of the nineteenth century. In the spring of 1881 one popular French journalist wrote, "The illness of our age is hysteria. One encounters it everywhere. Everywhere one rubs elbows with it. . . . Studying hysteria, Monsieur Laségue, the illustrious master, and Monsieur Charcot have put their finger on the wound of the day. . . . This singular neurosis with its astonishing effects . . . travels the streets and the world."

Although self-starvation resulting from stomach pain, lack of appetite, vomiting, or the sensation of having a lump in the throat began as a bit player in the grand drama of hysteria, it steadily gained prominence in the ranks of hysterical symptoms in the second half of the century. By 1860 Louis-Victor Marce, the director of a large asylum in France, reported that it was "very common" to observe "young women who, just having reached puberty after a precocious physical development, lose their appetite to an extreme degree. No matter how long they have abstained from food, they experience a distaste for it which even the most insistent urging is unable to reverse." Between 1860 and 1864 the young women in a Lisbon school alternated in groups between symptoms of hysteria—leg weakness, paralysis, and day blindness—and periods of vomiting that went on for months. At one point 90 out of 114 girls participated in the epidemic of vomiting.

As eating disordered behavior became increasingly common among hysterics, doctors began to debate its meaning and cause. Various labels appeared in the early literature, all hinting at different root causes: "apepsia hysterica," "neuropathic disorders of gastric sensibility," "nervous dyspepsia," "hyperaesthesias of the stomach," "gastrodynia," and "visceral neurosis." "In the years before the phenomenon received a formal diagnostic label," Shorter writes, "the symptoms tended to be inchoate and poorly defined because neither doctors nor patients had yet a clear model of the disease." This time of uncertainty, Shorter suggests, made for a kind of incubation period for the illness of anorexia, a time when the debates among doctors began to shape the public's and the patients' understanding of the behavior.

It wasn't until 1873 that anorexia nervosa finally received that formal recognition. That year Laségue, already famous for his work with hysterical patients, dubbed the disease "hysterical anorexia." (A year later the word "hysterical" would be dropped and the term "anorexia nervosa" would become standard in the medical literature.) The typical patient, he reported, was a young woman between 15 and 20 who had recently suffered an emotional trauma and began a "refusal of food that may be indefinitely prolonged." He noted that months might go by without the patient's health declining. Indeed she might enjoy a surge of energy. "Not only does she not sigh for recovery, but she is not ill pleased with her condition, notwithstanding the unpleasantness it is attended with."

For another historical scholar, the moment in time when a disease became officially recognized and named by the established medical order might be nothing more than an interesting historical footnote. Shorter, however, was an expert in the history of psychosomatic illnesses, and he knew better than anyone that the pronouncements of famous doctors could have a powerful, though unconscious, effect on people. As his body of research shows, history was full of ever-changing psychosomatic symptoms shaped in large part by the expectations and beliefs of the current medical establishment. "As doctors' own ideas about what constitutes 'real' disease change from time to time due to theory and practice, the symptoms that patients present will change as well," he writes. "These medical changes give the story of psychosomatic illness its dynamic: the medical 'shaping' of symptoms."

Shorter believes that it was Laségue's famous paper and the public interest in the medical debate surrounding the diagnosis of anorexia that forged a kind of template for self-starvation. As the medical establishment settled on the name, the agreed-upon causes, and a specific symptom list for the disease, they were, Shorter argues, "disseminating a model of how the patient was to behave and the doctor to respond." What was once a mishmash of conflicting medical theories surrounding self-starvation had now gained the appearance of a precise disorder with a specific at-risk population.

That new conception of this illness took hold not only among women who had already manifested disordered eating but in the population at large. There are no broad epidemiologic studies of eating disorders from the time, but the anecdotal evidence for what happened next is persuasive: soon after the official designation of anorexia nervosa, the incidence of the disease began a dramatic climb. Whereas in the 1850s self-starvation was a rare symptom associated with hysterics, by the end of the century the medical literature was littered with references to full-blown anorexics. As one London doctor reported in 1888, anorexic behavior was "a very common occurrence," of which he had "abundant opportunities of seeing and treating many interesting cases." In that same year a young medical student confidently wrote in his doctoral dissertation, "Among hysterics, nothing is more common than anorexia."

A New Behavior Dives into the Symptom Pool

What caused the increase in cases of anorexia in the late nineteenth century? Does the naming of a disorder allow doctors to suddenly recognize and report what they had previously overlooked? Or is there an interplay between the codification of a new mental illness and the sudden appearance of those symptoms in the general population? With the introduction of any new illness category (as we'll see in the chapters on depression in Japan and PTSD in Sri Lanka), there are always those who argue that the apparent increased incidence of a condition is simply due to the fact that the disease in question had previously gone unnoticed or underreported. Although there is often some truth to that assertion, the other possibility has rarely been squarely addressed. For his part, Shorter unequivocally argues that there is a clear connection between the official recognition of anorexia nervosa and the growing number of women who began to self-starve in Europe and then the United States.

Shorter believes that psychosomatic illnesses (such as leg paralysis at the turn of the twentieth century or multiple personality disorder at the turn of the twenty-first) are examples of the unconscious mind attempting to speak in a language of emotional distress that will be understood in its time. People at a given moment in history in need of expressing their psychological suffering have a limited number of symptoms to choose from—a "symptom pool," as he calls it. When someone unconsciously latches onto a behavior in the symptom pool, he or she is doing so for a very specific reason: the person is taking troubling emotions and internal conflicts that are often indistinct or frustratingly beyond expression and distilling them into a symptom or behavior that is a culturally recognized signal of suffering. "Patients unconsciously endeavor to produce symptoms that will correspond to the medical diagnostics of the time," Shorter told me when I called him in Montreal to speak with him about Lee's work. "This sort of cultural molding of the unconscious happens imperceptibly and follows a large number of cultural cues that patients simply are not aware of."

Because the patient is unconsciously striving for recognition and legitimization of internal distress, his or her subconscious will be drawn toward those symptoms that will achieve those ends. Such a dynamic makes the official public naming of a disease such as anorexia nervosa a perilous event. It is clear to Shorter that psychiatrists and physicians themselves have long been key players in validating which new disorders or behaviors appear in the symptom pool.

In the late nineteenth century the process of adding a new symptom to the hysteria symptom pool would go like this: On the basis of a few new and exciting cases, doctors would publicly describe and debate and then codify the new pathological behavior. Popular magazines, newspapers, and journals would write about the new medical findings. Women in the general population would unconsciously begin to manifest the behavior and seek help. Patients and doctors would then engage in what is called "illness negotiation," whereby they would together shape each other's perceptions of the behavior. In this negotiation the doctor would provide scientific validation that the symptom was indeed indicative of a legitimate disease category, and new patients would increase the attention focused on the new symptom in the professional and popular press, creating a feedback loop that further established the legitimacy of the new symptom.

So although there may have been a small number of patients who presented novel behaviors without a cultural template (like Lee's atypical anorexics in Hong Kong), the widespread adoption of a new hysterical symptom such as anorexia or leg paralysis would *follow* the official "discovery" of the symptom or disorder and the establishment of the cultural feedback loop.

Anorexia was rare in the mid-nineteenth century not because physicians somehow failed to notice their starving patients, Shorter believes, but because it hadn't yet been widely acknowledged as part of the symptom pool of that time. Only after it became a culturally agreed-upon expression of internal distress did it become widespread.

Interestingly, pathological behaviors don't attain a permanent place in the symptom pool. It takes a certain amount of public and professional attention to keep behaviors like those common to hysteria in play in the minds of a population. And indeed in the middle part of the twentieth century many of the most dramatic symptoms connected to hysteria drifted out of the symptom pool. When the psychiatrist Hilde Bruch began her study of anorexia in the 1940s, she reported that it was once again "so rare . . . that it was practically unknown." Searching the admissions records at Presbyterian Hospital in New York during those middle decades of the twentieth century, she found on average only one case per year. Like Lee's anorexics, the patients Bruch saw during those years often weren't aware that their condition had a name, nor did they know others who suffered similarly. Each one, she recalls, "was an original inventor of this effort at self-assertion." The disorder once again became the topic of intense public and professional interest after February 4, 1983, when the popular singer Karen Carpenter collapsed from heart failure brought on by anorexia nervosa. After that jump in interest, the number of articles on the topic steadily grew throughout the decade. By the late 1980s you'd have been hard-pressed to find a Western teenager, especially among those girls in the high-achieving, upper-middle-class demographic group, who did not know about anorexia nervosa. It was back in the symptom pool, luring another generation of women.

A Clean Slate

Looking at the rise and fall and rise of anorexia over the century, Lee was convinced, like Shorter, that eating disorders were not at all like diseases such as the mumps or polio; they didn't have a natural history that could be separated from the specific time and place in which they existed. "Mental illnesses, specifically anorexia, do not exist independent of social and historical context," Lee concluded. "There may therefore be no true natural history of [anorexia nervosa], but rather a social history at a given time and place, a perspective which questions radically the biomedical assumption that there is a 'core problem' with [anorexia nervosa]."

Lee began to suspect that his handful of atypical cases in Hong Kong were akin to the rare cases of self-starvation in the early nineteenth century, before it had been codified by the prominent psychiatrists and physicians of the day and publicized around the Western world. "I began to think that these atypical patients I was seeing might shed some light on the early appearance of self-starvation before it became known as anorexia," he recalls. "You can't go back a hundred or two hundred years to re-interview early anorexic patients."

He came to believe that the reason his patients didn't report their self-starvation as coming from a fear of fatness was because that explanation would have made no sense in their cultural surroundings. Fear of fatness wasn't recognized in the Hong Kong culture as a legitimate reason for self-starvation; it was therefore unavailable to the patient both as a private belief and as an explanation she might give her doctor.

However, there were other explanations at the time that did make sense. For instance, the Chinese have historically looked to bodily sensations to indicate psychological distress. Because of this long history of somaticizing mental distress, it made sense to Lee that the atypical anorexics he was seeing often focused on stomach complaints and the feeling of bloating as the cause of their behavior. Chinese philosophical thinking avoided making the Cartesian distinction between the mind and the body. A Chinese girl's complaint of stomach pain might carry as much meaning and impact as a signal of emotional distress as a Western teenager's complaint of anxiety or depression. Lee also saw in his patients echoes of a certain Confucian asceticism—an almost monk-like self-denial, asexuality, and lack of worry about their bodily decline or even death. "Their food denial communicated powerful cultural symbols, private meanings and interpersonal messages," Lee concluded. Decoding these messages required a deep understanding of the specific cultural forces influencing the self-conception of these women.

In trying to parse out these meanings, Lee was racing against time. Even as he was making progress understanding the particular cultural meanings behind food refusal in Hong Kong, the Western diagnosis of anorexia was becoming accepted across the globe. Lee feared that the *DSM* diagnosis of anorexia, with its focus on fat phobia and body image distortion, would obscure more subtle, culturally specific forms of self-starvation.

Slowly but steadily, in the early 1990s he noticed mental health providers around him succumbing to a kind of color-blindness, an inability to see the cultural and individual differences in the patients they interviewed. As each year passed, he could see the influence of the Western diagnostic manual grow, particularly in younger generations of clinicians. Reviewing other doctors' notes on new cases of anorexia referred to him, he would see such sentences as "The patient still denied having a fear of fatness or dieting." For these younger doctors, it couldn't be a case of anorexia unless it conformed to the *DSM* criteria. Lee worried that these clinicians were adhering to a foreign diagnostic manual at the expense of understanding both the patient's subjective experience and the cultural meaning specific to Hong Kong at that time. If they became blind to the local realities of their patients, he feared, they would have little hope in treating them.

A Death on Wan Chai Road

Although the psychologists and psychiatrists in Hong Kong began to adopt the *DSM* description of anorexia, the general population of Hong Kong remained largely unaware of the disease. As of the early 1990s, there had yet to be any outreach campaigns to local high schools. There had been no Chinese celebrities afflicted with the disorder and little reported about the condition in newspaper or magazine articles.

Lee speculated that this very lack of public awareness about anorexia might be key to the rarity of the disorder, reducing the likelihood that distressed individuals would choose, as he put it, "anorexia as a convenient form of illness." Which is another way of saying that anorexia remained outside the symptom pool for the majority of the population. Lee had a fear, though. As he wrote prophetically in 1989, he worried that somewhere there might be an "epidemiogenic trigger" for anorexia that, once tripped, would "exert an explosive effect." Five years later that fear was realized.

At 1 p.m. on November 24, 1994, the last day of her life, 14-year-old Charlene Hsu Chi-Ying walked past the trophy case at Saint Paul Secondary School, underneath the banner of the Virgin Mary, and out into the Happy Valley district of Hong Kong. Wearing her school uniform and carrying her school backpack, she was unsteady on her feet. She had fainted twice in the previous week. Just the day before, she had blacked out in front of her school and had to be sent to the nurse's office with a cut knee.

Heading home from Happy Valley to her family's apartment in the Healthy Gardens high-rise complex, she walked north through a forest of skyscrapers toward the central business district of Hong Kong. Having grown up in the city, she found the cultural mélange she passed through to be quite normal. She passed the Seventh Day

Adventist Pioneer Memorial Church and a Buddhist temple. She walked by one McDonald's and another a few blocks later. She walked past the Hong Kong Cemetery, the Saint Michael Catholic Cemetery, and then past the Muslim cemetery. She also passed by the front doors of the hospital where her lifeless body would soon be delivered.

Charlene was about to become famous in Hong Kong as the public face of anorexia nervosa. Her death that day would introduce the disorder into the public consciousness and be a critical turning point in the evolution and spread of the illness. It is therefore important to try to understand—both intellectually and on a gut level—what it meant to be a 14-year-old in Hong Kong at that particular moment in history.

The mid-1990s were an uncertain and nervous time for the population of Hong Kong. The transfer of sovereignty from Britain to China was just three years away. Even before the 1989 Tiananmen Square protests, many families had attempted to emigrate. After the massacre the number of those trying to get out of Hong Kong doubled; before the handover more than half a million people would leave.

This caused a great deal of stress on family networks. Most countries allowed families to immigrate only in Western-style nuclear groups: a set of parents and a set of children. But traditional Chinese ties to extended families remained strong. Indeed in the unforgiving and competitive business environment of Hong Kong, support from extended families was an important social safety net. The emigration of each family unit weakened that safety net for the relatives left behind.

"Through the early 1990s, each time we returned from summer holidays, a few more children had disappeared to Canada, Australia, the United States, Britain," wrote one of Charlene's contemporaries. "For us confused adolescents, it was a blur of hasty farewells to friends pulled out of school midterm. . . . All around us, people were panicking about the future of the British colony, stunned by the bloody crushing of the student-led protests in Beijing."

One can get a sense of the confluence of these forces in the Hong Kong of the 1990s by watching movies about teen life during the period. One in particular, *Autumn Moon,* directed by Clara Law in 1992, tells us a great deal. Along with those of other so-called second-wave directors in Hong Kong, Law's films are moody and strive to communicate the postmodern disconnect of the time. *Autumn Moon* is about a 15-year-old Hong Kong girl who strikes up an unlikely friendship with a bored and nihilistic Japanese tourist named Tokio. The teenage girl, Hui, is caught between two countries: her parents have already emigrated to Canada, leaving her in Hong Kong to wait for the death of her grandmother. Like Tokio, Hui is disconnected from traditional culture. She can't cook and believes that McDonald's represents traditional Chinese food. The movie also riffs on the globalization of teen culture; when Hui worries that in Canada no one will have heard of Madonna, Tokio reassures her, "Don't worry. Madonna is everywhere."

As the movie suggests, no segment of the world's population is more vulnerable to being swept away by the currents of globalization than adolescents. Teenagers are often the first to adopt Western dress and slang and identify with movies, music, and television. But *Autumn Moon* reveals that teenagers in Hong Kong were not simply interested in Western pop cultural tastes in music and food. What was changing was the very nature of adolescence. The first scene shows Hui standing in front of her bedroom mirror; in a voiceover she says, "I am fifteen years old. I've only just found out that the cold weather doesn't start right after summer. Autumn is in between."

Social scientists have coined a shorthand for the Western view of adolescence, calling it "storm and stress." Research in the United

States and Europe has consistently shown that the teenage years bring with them the highest prevalence of risky behavior, including substance abuse, wild driving, and unprotected sex. Some researchers have assumed that what we've learned about adolescence in the United States and Europe is true of teenagers around the world.

Cross-cultural research has shown, however, that the storm and stress assumptions about adolescence are far from universal. According to Jeffrey Jensen Arnett, a professor at Clark University and the author of *Adolescence and Emerging Adulthood: A Cultural Approach*, at the heart of the cross-cultural difference is the importance placed on achieving independence. Our Western conception of adulthood places a high value on individual identity and self-sufficiency, and much of the storm and stress of Western adolescence comes from the push and pull of this movement toward separation.

However, in many traditional cultures, particularly in Asia, personal independence has not been the goal of adulthood. Instead, *inter*dependence—reliance on and obedience to one's family, clan, and village—has been the goal. Teenagers on their path to adulthood are not expected to strain the bonds that tie them to their family. Because traditional cultures have de-emphasized the notion that adolescence is the road to personal independence, much of the storm and stress experienced by Western adolescents has been absent.

But there were signs that this was changing. "If it is true that cultural values of individualism lie at the heart of adolescent storm and stress," Arnett concludes, "it seems likely that adolescence in traditional cultures will become more stormy and stressful . . . as the influence of the West increases."

So not only were governmental and family structures undergoing rapid change in the mid-1990s in Hong Kong, but the very nature of adolescence was in flux. Social stress on the adolescent population was obvious; what had yet to be determined was how that inchoate psychological charge would express itself.

Thinner Than a Yellow Flower

It was during this nervous time in the history of Hong Kong that Charlene Hsu Chi-Ying began to lose weight. Until late in the summer of 1994 she had been a parent's dream. Her grades and test scores consistently put her in the top percentile of her school. She had a close group of friends and was active in sports and afterschool activities. Her mother was never sure why her daughter started to eat less, as the incident that seemed to spark her food refusal seemed trivial: her mother had not let her go on a class trip to mainland China.

Once her weight loss started in August, her personality quickly changed as well. By October she had become sullen and uncommunicative. She never mentioned that she was trying to diet, nor did she mention believing that she was overweight. Her classmates noticed the change in her personality. Once a gregarious girl with a group of friends, by October of that school year she had taken to sitting in the corner of the lunch room by herself, reading while the other students ate.

Although the diagnosis of anorexia never came up, both a school counselor and an outside social worker met with Charlene to encourage her to eat more and go to a doctor for a checkup. The last meeting with school personnel took place the day she fainted in front of the school. The schoolmistress, Ting Yi, said that the staff had decided not to tell Charlene's parents about the incident but to use the threat as leverage for change. Charlene had one week, they told her, to improve herself before they would notify her parents.

The next day Charlene took her fateful last walk. After passing by the graveyards and the hospital, she turned onto the busy Wan Chai Road. This is where she often hopped a tram to take her home to Healthy Gardens. Before she reached the tram stop she became unsteady on her feet. A shopkeeper from across the street named Chan Suk-kuen spotted Charlene. She would later tell the inquest board that Charlene caught her attention because she was so preternaturally thin. The shopkeeper briefly lost sight of her when a double-decker tram obscured her from view. When the tram passed, she saw that Charlene had collapsed onto the sidewalk. Chan Suk-kuen and half a dozen other people came to her aid. When she didn't revive, they called the police and an ambulance.

The policeman who checked her backpack and found her school identification card at first couldn't reconcile the smiling and healthy young woman in the picture with the emaciated and ghostly figure being loaded onto a gurney. The coroner who examined Charlene's body, Dr. Au Kam-wah, found that she weighed 75 pounds. Her adrenal gland, thyroid, kidney, and stomach all showed signs of atrophy. She had virtually no stores of subcutaneous fat. Her heart was tiny, weighing just three ounces. The policeman's confusion was repeated at the hospital, where several of the nurses, upon seeing the skeletal body on the stretcher, initially assumed it was the remains of an elderly woman.

Had Charlene made it home and died in her family's apartment in Healthy Gardens, her passing might not have caught the attention of the media. However, because she collapsed on a busy shopping street in the heart of Hong Kong, the story was irresistible. All of Hong Kong's Chinese and English papers gave prominent placement to the story of her death. "School Girl Falls on Ground Dead: Anorexia Made Her Skin and Bones," read one headline in a Chinese-language paper. "Girl Who Died in Street Was a Walking Skeleton," reported the English-language *South China Morn-*

ing Post. "Schoolgirl Falls Dead on Street: Thinner Than a Yellow Flower," reported another Chinese-language daily.

The Chinese-language papers used the phrase *yan shi zheng* for the disorder. *Yan* means to loathe or to dislike, *shi* means eating, and *zheng* means disease or disorder. The literal translation of the term for anorexia in both the Cantonese and Mandarin dialects would be something along the lines of "the disorder of loathing to eat" or "the disease of disliking eating." This was the first time people in Hong Kong had read about a local case of anorexia in their daily papers.

Of course all of the articles tried to address the burning question on everyone's mind: What was the meaning behind this strange disease that led a young girl to starve herself to death?

To answer the question, Chinese reporters looked to Western sources and experts. One reporter for a Chinese-language daily was clearly cribbing from the *DSM* when he described anorexia this way: "The patients are so afraid of gaining weight, that even when they are underweight, they insist that they are fat." Several papers quoted Western experts to explain that dieting and the fashion industry were culpable. "Weight loss became a tragedy!" began one story. "It was speculated that a 15-year-old girl had been losing weight with the wrong methods, and her health condition deteriorated day by day." Dieting and the beauty industry were not the only causes cited in the papers. "Besides weight loss for beauty, other causes of anorexia include family strife and school pressure," claimed one article in a Chinese-language daily. It also noted that the pressure of being a celebrity sometimes brings on the disorder, reminding readers that a famous American singer had died of the disease.

A year later a public inquest was held to determine the cause of Charlene's death. Charlene's mother, schoolmates, teachers, and counselors all gave testimony. The papers ran stories emphasizing that anorexia nervosa was a dangerous disease that threatened young women in Hong Kong. Headlines read "Call for Vigilance to Prevent Anorexia Deaths" and "Teen Death Sparks Anorexia Concern."

There was no evidence at that moment that anorexia was a widespread disorder among young women in Hong Kong. Indeed the tone of alarm in the headlines and the leads of the stories was often contradicted by quotes from local experts near the bottom of the story. On the stand, the pathologist Dr. Au Kam-wah testified that he had seen only one other possible case of anorexia in his ten years of practice. Nevertheless the jury at the inquest recommended that schools provide counseling and education on eating disorders and their consequences. The papers followed suit. "Teachers, social workers, parents and schoolmates should make a combined effort to detect anorexia among secondary school girls before it is too late," began one follow-up story in *The Standard*.

Lies about Beauty

It is difficult to document when a psychosomatic symptom such as self-starvation worms its way into the unconscious minds of a population. There is, of course, no single moment when a behavior enters the symptom pool of a culture. Looking back over time, however, it is often possible to identify a tipping point, the period after which the public's knowledge and acceptance of a symptom or disorder begins to grow exponentially. There is little doubt that the year of Charlene's death represented that crucial tipping point for anorexia in Hong Kong.

The day before I visited Dr. Lee during my visit to Hong Kong, I spent an afternoon flipping through the press clipping files of the Hong Kong Eating Disorders Association with the organization's clinical psychologist, Celia Wu. The popular press articles that were published about anorexia after 1994 were remarkable both in their volume and in how similar they were to Western popular press articles on the topic. Within a few years of Charlene's death, there were several Hong Kong actresses and pop singers telling harrowing stories of becoming anorexic. In one article Western celebrity anorexics were compared side-by-side with their Hong Kong counterparts.

The cultural trends identified as the cause of the disorder were familiar as well. "Swallowing Lies about Beauty Can Make You Sick," read a headline in *The Standard* in 1995. "Western influence," the article claims, "brings with it the notion of 'happy go skinny.' Supermodels on catwalks, Hollywood stars at the Oscars, and even the slender legs in beer and automobile adverts all promote the anorexic look as sexy and glamorous." "Teenagers Risk Health in Quest for Beauty: Expert Blames Social Pressures for Eating Disorders as Patient Numbers Soar," read another typical headline.

Remarkably, the pieces in both Chinese-language and English-language papers often relied exclusively on Western psychologists and psychiatrists to explain the illness. The Western experts quoted in these popular articles repeated variations on the common themes that dieting and pop cultural trends caused anorexia and that fear of being fat was central to the illness. None suggested that there might be meaningful distinctions between the manifestation of anorexia in the West and East.

Quoting Western sources, the media coverage in Hong Kong repeated several ideas, including the following:

- That anorexia was a threat to young women who were prone to anxiety or depression or facing problems in school or in their families.

- That severe food restriction in young women should be read as a cry for help.

- That a key spark for the disorder lay in shifting cultural ideas of thinness and beauty.

- That fat phobia and a distorted body image defined the disorder.

- That anorexia usually attacked the most promising young women.

This conception of anorexia mirrors fairly well the understanding one would find in the West among educated people and non–eating disorder specialists in the medical and mental health fields.* The idea that anorexia is tied to culturally imposed notions of female beauty has become conventional wisdom in the West. "In casual conversation we hear this idea expressed all the time: Anorexia is caused by the incessant drumbeat of modern dieting, by the erotic veneration of sylphlike women," writes Joan Jacobs Brumberg in her masterpiece *Fasting Girls: The History of Anorexia Nervosa.*

The problem was that many of these Western assumptions had little meaning for most of the anorexics Lee saw in his practice. Those women were not motivated by ideas of thinness and beauty. They were not fat phobic, nor did they have a distorted body image. They were not the "golden girls" of their schools or workplace. The mental health experts quoted in the Hong Kong papers and magazines confidently reported that anorexia in Hong Kong was the same disorder that appeared in the United States and Europe. In Lee's experience, this was simply not the case.

---

*Not that an eating disorder specialist would necessarily disagree with these items. I mean to point out only that the Western research literature on anorexia goes far beyond these baseline assumptions in both complexity and diversity of opinion. What was being transmitted to Hong Kong in the mid-1990s, in other words, was a lay Westerner's view of anorexia, the sort of information you'd glean if you read about anorexia in a weekly news magazine.

Western assumptions about the disease were spread not only through the popular press and television. Western academic researchers also took up the charge. Shirley Geok-Lin Lim, a professor of English at the University of California, Santa Barbara and a visiting professor at the University of Hong Kong, wrote in the journal *American Studies International* that the rise in anorexia in Hong Kong was due to a "globalization of a visual culture in which women's bodies and appearances are homogenized and fetishized as childlike or waif-like, subordinate and vulnerable."

Although Lee was trained in the West, his frustration at this lopsided emphasis on Western knowledge when it came to anorexia sometimes boiled over. "It is sobering to recognize that although the non-Western cultures are sub-dominant and ill-prepared to publish, they make up 80% of the world," Lee wrote testily in an article published in 1995. Indeed the unthinking adoption of the *DSM* diagnosis of anorexia threatened to turn the very act of disease labeling into a meaningless abstraction, one that could harm the doctor-patient relationship by blinding them both to the more subtle and complex realities of the patient's history and her local experience of culture. Lee wrote, "By intentionally replacing native metaphors with experience-distancing jargons and by unintentionally demolishing cultures, the imposition of universalizing biomedical categories may imperil illness negotiation on the one hand, and curtail local healing opportunities on the other."

Lee's effort to alert the world to the important differences in local expressions of anorexia in Hong Kong did not go unheard, at least within the community of those who seriously study eating disorders. Beginning with his early research, his papers on the topic appeared in the top international journals and received wide praise from other scholars. But in terms of influencing the general population's understanding of the meaning of anorexia, Lee's work appeared to have little effect.

In the wake of Charlene's death educational programs were launched in schools, further spreading news of the disorder. A youth support organization called Kids Everywhere Like You (KELY) announced that it was going to set up special counseling programs to focus on the threat of eating disorders. They also announced a twenty-four-hour hotline in both English and Cantonese to provide information and counseling.

All these avenues for information fed the general public's understanding of the disease. Hong Kong teenagers became increasingly aware that eating disorders were no longer a Western phenomenon. They now understood that they were at risk as well.

What happened over the next few years mirrors what happened in the United States and Europe after the naming of the disease. As the public became aware that anorexia was in the symptom pool, local clinicians, including Lee, noticed an increase in cases of eating disorders. Where Lee was once seeing two or three anorexic patients a year, he was now seeing that many new cases each week. The increase sparked a new series of newspaper, magazine, and television reports. One typical article noted that eating disorders were "twice as common as shown in earlier studies and that the incidence is increasing rapidly." In the late 1990s, studies reported that between 3 and 10 percent of young women in Hong Kong showed disordered eating behavior. "Children as Young as 10 Starving Themselves as Eating Ailments Rise," announced a headline in *The Standard*. The lead stated: "A university yesterday produced figures showing a 25-fold increase in cases of such disorders."

Amid all the finger-pointing at diet fads and the influence of Western fashion and pop culture, few considered the possibility that the idea of anorexia nervosa itself—prepackaged in its *DSM* diagnosis and explained by readily available Western experts—might have been part of the reason the disorder caught on so quickly in Hong Kong. This possibility, however, fits well with Shorter's theory of how symptom pools change over time. At another point in history, the population of troubled teenage girls might be drawn to a different unconscious behavior to express their internal distress. But starting in 1994 a new belief became prominent in the culture of Hong Kong. Each newspaper article, magazine essay, and television show that depicted anorexia as a valid and dramatic expression of mental distress for young women made that conclusion self-fulfilling. Each repetition of this idea incrementally increased the gravitational pull of the disorder on the unconscious minds of the population, making it ever more likely that a teenager would try food restriction as a method of communicating her internal distress. The greater the number of women who experienced the symptom, the more public concern and media attention was directed toward the disease.

Of course, over time a public interest in disordered eating might have evolved in Hong Kong without Western ideas. The critical question is, however, Would the cultural feedback loop have spun into motion so quickly without the importation of the Western template for the disease? It seems unlikely. Beginning with the scattered European cases in the early nineteenth century, it took more than fifty years for the disease to be named, categorized, and popularized by Western mental health professionals. By contrast, after Charlene fell onto the sidewalk on Wan Chai Road on November 24, 1994, it was just a matter of hours before the Hong Kong population learned the name of the disease, who was at risk, and what it meant. The people of Hong Kong did not come to these conclusions without help. Rather, they imported the meaning of anorexia from the West—no assembly required.

"Me-Too" Anorexics

The increase in cases of the disorder was not the only remarkable thing that happened after Charlene's death. At the same time that Lee was trying to alert the world that anorexia in Hong Kong had its own distinct expression, the disease presentation among young women in Hong Kong began to change.

A survey of adolescent anorexics between 1992 and 1997 showed a clear shift in the anorexic patients' explanation for their behavior. Unlike Lee's earlier patients, by 1997 fat phobia had become the single most important reason given for their self-starvation. Eighty percent of these young eating disordered patients, in fact, said that their key reason for self-starvation was the fear of becoming fat. By 2007 almost all the anorexics he treated reported fat phobia. New patients were increasingly conforming their experience of anorexia to the Western version of the disease.

Were doctors and patients reporting fat phobia and body image distortion simply to put the condition in line with the *DSM?* Lee believes the shifting social understanding of anorexia actually influenced the expression of the disease on the deeper level of the patient's experience. Patients were not simply reporting fat phobia and body image distortion but actually experiencing those symptoms. Aspects of the disease seen in Lee's early patients, such as the feeling of fullness or bloating in the stomach, lost their cultural salience, their ability to communicate internal distress. The importation of the Western diagnosis was not only changing the way patients and doctors talked about the disorder—it was changing the disease experience itself.

Lee came to believe that there are basically two populations from which eating disordered patients come. A small percentage begin to self-starve on their own. These women unconsciously choose self-starvation because of some set of experiences and unconscious currents that are unique to their particular lives. (It is likely, he believes, that there have been a small number of self-styled anorexics throughout history.) These are the sorts of patients that Shorter wrote about from the mid-nineteenth century and Bruch saw in the 1940s.

But at different moments in history there arises another population of eating disordered patients; they come to the behavior with a cultural understanding of how it is acted out, who is at risk, and what attitudes and behaviors result from the condition. The "holy anorexics" of late medieval times would fall into this category, as would those women with hysteria in the late nineteenth century.

Bruch saw the distinction between these two groups during her research. The rare anorexic patient she met in 1940s New York, she reports, was distinct from the dozens of young anorexic women she treated starting in the 1970s. "Those who had developed the illness during the 1970s often had 'known' about the illness, or even knew someone who had it . . . [or] deliberately 'tried it out' after having watched a TV program," she wrote in one of her final papers before her death in 1984. "Instead of the fierce search for independence [which defined earlier patients] these 'me-too' anorexics compete with or cling to each other."

The different characteristics of these two groups are interesting but less important than another fact: the women attracted to the disorder when there exists a cultural template for the behavior inevitably far outnumber the women who come to food restriction on their own. Once an eating disorder becomes an accepted "pattern of misconduct," Richard Gordon writes in *Eating Disorders: Anatomy of a Social Epidemic*, "individuals with pre-existing mood or anxiety disorders, or a whole host of underlying psychopathologies or developmental vulnerabilities, histories of sexual abuse or familial concerns with weight control, may be predisposed to adopting such culturally sanctioned behaviors as modes of managing unbearable levels of distress."

The patients Lee documented in the second half of the 1990s appeared to be mostly of the "me-too" type. Lee believes that stress from the rapid social changes occurring in Hong Kong led to a "general loading of psychopathology" within the population. At such moments there is no universal way for psychological distress to express itself; the manifestation of such stress reflects the symptom pool of the time. Once the idiom of eating disorders became understood, many of these young women used the behavior to express their inchoate anxiety and unhappiness. "When there is a cultural atmosphere in which professionals, the media, schools, doctors, psychologists all recognize and endorse and talk about and publicize eating disorders," Lee explains, "then people with a certain loading of this general psychopathology can be triggered to consciously or unconsciously pick eating disorder pathology as a way to express that conflict."

As if to prove the point that eating disorders can act like contagions that blow across national boundaries on the cultural currents, the late 1990s saw the rapid rise of another type of eating disorder. In late 1995 Princess Diana gave her famous interview confirming the rumors that she had suffered from bulimia for more than four years. "You inflict it upon yourself because your self-esteem is at a low ebb, and you don't think you're worthy or valuable," she said during the interview, which was carried on Hong Kong television and widely discussed in the press. "I was crying out for help." The newspapers again blared headlines warning about the new disorder.

Once again an eating disorder symptom had arrived in Hong Kong's symptom pool with cultural momentum it had gained elsewhere. Purging behaviors, including self-induced vomiting and the use of laxatives and diuretics, quickly spread among the adolescent population. Patients themselves often reported to their doctors that the impetus to try these techniques came from reading or hearing about others with the disorder. Although dieting was usually the expressed goal, it was hearing or reading about bulimia itself that was often the spark for the pathological behavior. "In line with trends witnessed in Western countries," Lee wrote at the time, "bulimia is likely to become an increasingly 'fashionable' mode of coping with distress among young Chinese women in the coming decade."

Meeting an Atypical Anorexic

In 1907 Picasso created a painting of five nude women he titled *Les Demoiselles d'Avignon*. Now famous for being an early work of the cubist period that was about to blossom in Paris, the painting is initially disorienting. Each of the women's figures is distorted in some manner: breasts and elbows are at sharp angles, feet and arms are out of proportion compared to heads; the faces of two of the women depicted on the left of the painting look like African masks. The painting has a strange mismatch of styles, at once representative, impressionistic, and abstract.

Melanie Katzman, a feminist medical scholar from Cornell Medical School, and Sing Lee wrote about that painting in a joint paper they published in 1997. In their view, the image is a metaphor for the approach that must be taken when trying to understand women suffering from eating disorders in general and anorexia nervosa in particular. Just as Picasso used different artistic styles to depict his subjects, the meaning behind eating disorders can be understood only when approached cross-disciplinarily. This would be tragic, they argued, if researchers failed to see the cross-cultural differences in anorexic behavior and instead put all such women in a Western mold. Katzman and Lee were writing not just of what had happened in Hong Kong. In Tokyo, Singapore, Cape Town, and Jerusalem the discovery of eating disorders was quickly followed by the arrival of American-made knowledge that defined what an eating disorder was and what it meant.

Katzman and Lee hoped that mental health professionals would "break through the constraints of current 'bodily obsessed analysis' in which fat phobia and body image distortion are esteemed as the universal driving force behind food refusal." The *DSM* version of the disorder was obscuring the indigenous distresses and patterns of behavior that led young women to adopt self-starvation. If clinicians around the world could avoid the quick and easy adoption of Western assumptions about anorexia, they might be able to hear the complex truths individual women were trying to communicate. Anorexia and eating disorders could tell us much about the pressures on women in different cultures if only their voices weren't being drowned out by Western narratives about the power of fashion, dieting, and pop culture.

Wanting me to understand this point on a personal level, Lee let me spend an afternoon with one of his long-term patients whom I'll call Ling. I knew something about Ling before I met her; Lee had written about her case prominently over the years.

During our interview, which was facilitated by a translator, Ling stayed bundled in an oversized ski jacket with a Pink Panther logo. Even so, it was clear from her frail hands and the prominent tendons in her neck that she was seriously underweight. Throughout our interview she sat almost perfectly still, with her hands clasped in her lap and her knees held tightly together. Her expression was sad, and she often looked at the floor while she talked.

Ling had grown up in an unhappy lower-class family. Her father, who worked off and on as a glass cutter, was a bad-tempered alcoholic who violently abused his wife and children. Ling told me that her father had sexually fondled her on several occasions when she was 12. Not surprisingly, she hated him and secretly fantasized about his death. She had repeated nightmares in which she was weeping and running away from her father as he "chased her like the devil."

Ling's troubles with food began at the dinner table, where her siblings, her mother, and she had to tolerate the angry and often drunken tirades of her father. To describe the experience of eating with her father she used the Chinese saying, "being forced to drink bitter tea." In hopes of getting the ordeal over as quickly as possible, she would sometimes bolt her food, willfully scalding the inside of her mouth. More often she simply found that she had no appetite when she sat down at the family table.

The second of four siblings, she had been plagued by feelings of insecurity and low self-esteem her entire life. When she was in her late teens and studying for her Hong Kong Certificate Examination she began to experience headaches and insomnia. Her menstrual cycle became irregular and then stopped altogether. She had stomach pains that were so intense that a doctor removed her appendix, but to no avail. Not surprisingly, she performed poorly on the test and had to quit school to take a job in a factory calculating wages. She cried often during this time and began to lose interest in everyone and everything around her, including eating. She made a halfhearted suicide attempt by drinking detergent. She tried to join a church but found her fellow worshippers no more kind or accepting than her coworkers or strangers on the subway. Ling led a life of utter social disconnection. For months she would go to work and then straight home, speaking to no one.

Like many anorexics of that time, she took a circuitous path to Lee's door. Her last stop in the medical system before Lee was to a gynecologist, where she was hoping to get help restarting her menstrual cycle. She admitted that this was her mother's concern more than her own. Her mother thought her lack of menstruation made her unsuitable for marriage. Ling herself had no interest in sex, marriage, or having children.

Lee first met Ling in 1992 when she was 29 years old. At that time she weighed 70 pounds, far below her ideal body weight of 101 pounds. He gave her a standard test used in the West to diagnose disordered eating behavior. From her answers it was clear that Ling did not fit the Western conception of anorexia.

When Ling first became aware that there was a disease category called anorexia, she couldn't see how it applied to her. From her perspective, her behavior wasn't focused on food. She protested that her problem was that her life lacked meaning. She didn't care about food in the same way she didn't care about her career or love life or maintaining social connections. If she didn't want to live, why would she be hungry?

While being treated by Lee in the early 1990s, she moved from her family home to the thirty-second floor of one of Hong Kong's many slender apartment high-rises. Even by Hong Kong standards she lived in a cramped space: less than 280 square feet. Her tiny bed was shorter than her height and she slept curled up. The bathtub was just three feet long. She often bruised herself while laundering clothes in the cramped bathroom. Living alone, she was something of a rebel. The tradition at the time for unmarried women in Hong Kong was to live with family.

In 2000, when her weight again dropped to 70 pounds, she was briefly hospitalized. By this time there were enough anorexics in Hong Kong that they had their own hospital ward. Meeting these other women, she again questioned her diagnosis. She learned that other anorexics misused laxatives and diuretics and were intentionally dieting to lose weight. "These behaviors sounded strange and awful to me," Ling told me. "I was not on a diet and I did not have a tendency of wanting to lose weight. I didn't have any of these behaviors, so I thought, 'I must not have this illness.'"

To this day Ling is still confused about what ails her. After meeting other anorexics and reading more about the disorder in the papers, she continues to wonder whether the disorder describes her condition. This reaction to the diagnosis, common among his atypical patients, has led Lee to ask a rather radical question: Is there any therapeutic value to categorizing patients such as Ling under one unifying disease label?

"You might want to group patients under a universal diagnosis if you faced a condition for which a particular drug had proved effective," Lee told me. "But there is no effective drug treatment for anorexia. The only meaningful components of treatment are understanding the patient's life and creating a motivation for the person to change. Does a medical diagnosis help with these goals? I am not convinced it does." A diagnosis such as anorexia, particularly if that diagnosis comes prepackaged with ideas and beliefs from a foreign land, can easily obscure the complex realities of the individual.

Ling, 44 when I interviewed her, expressed deep shame over a life she feels she has wasted and the burden she has caused her family. The one bright spot in life, she reported, was that she has begun to attend church again. "I feel it is important to have a religion," she told me. "I feel some motivation to do things now."

The Commodification of Anorexia

The rise of eating disorders in Hong Kong reveals an uncomfortable truth: our cultural fascination with the meaning of the eating disorders—our natural desire to understand the lesson behind them and alert the world to their danger—can become part of the feedback loop by which the disease goes forward and claims new victims. That there is a connection between public and professional attention to such disorders and their spread within a community is an idea that is only rarely whispered in the professional literature on the topic. Not surprisingly, popular book writers, researchers, and mental health educators are loath to see themselves as a vector transmitting the disease they hope to eradicate.

Regardless, it is important to look back at the recent increase in the number of cases of the disorder in the West and try to trace this effect. To begin with, there is no doubt that anorexia became iconic, a cause célèbre, within the feminist movement of the 1970s and 1980s. Whatever else can be said about the disorder, anorexia packs a wallop of a metaphoric punch. As the feminist philosopher Susan Bordo pointed out, anorexia calls attention to "the central ills of our culture." The disease has been endlessly employed to illustrate the social plight of women. In various writings on the topic, anorexia has been used to decry unrealistic body image standards, patriarchal family structures, the subjugation of women by postindustrial capitalism, unrealistic ideals of perfection, and more.

Unfortunately, in making these arguments writers have often unintentionally glamorized the disease and elevated the social role of the sufferer. Law professor Roberta Dresser argued in the *Wisconsin Law Review* in 1984 that medical and parental efforts to forcibly renourish anorexics should be challenged as a violation of the patient's civil liberties. She made the case that anorexics were similar to political hunger strikers, bravely challenging social injustice. They should be allowed to starve as a matter of free expression.

Joan Jacobs Brumberg, the feminist author of *Fasting Girls: The History of Anorexia Nervosa,* saw such "romanticization of anorexia" as deeply problematic, as did many of the most insightful feminist writers on the topic. She worried that the promotion of anorexia as a "protest against patriarchy" would overwhelm the more subtle and nonpolitical psychological realities of the women caught in the throes of the disease. "As a feminist," Blumberg writes, "I believe that the anorexic deserves our sympathy but not necessarily our veneration." Although it was seldom acknowledged, the worry behind such statements seems clear: veneration encourages imitation.

With the maturing of the feminist movement, this siren song to potential anorexics has largely died away. No recent feminist writers that I'm aware of have argued like Dresser that anorexics should be allowed to starve themselves to death to prove a political point. Still, anorexia and bulimia remain in the symptom pool of our time for more subtle and intractable reasons.

Those who devote their lives to treating disease are in a conundrum that has rarely gained public attention. At the same time that they are researching, publishing, and publicly speaking about these eating disorders, they are both molding the public's understanding of the behavior and keeping it in the symptom pool of our time. The South African psychologist Lesley Swartz is one of a very few who have addressed this difficult issue. "Regardless of the amount of care taken in education about any condition, professionals are inevitably involved in maintaining and shaping it," he writes. "We must allow that an environment receptive to the understanding of eating disorders may be one in which they will flourish."

Sometimes the extent to which researchers avoid this troubling issue is startling. A recent study by several British researchers showed a remarkable parallel between the incidence of bulimia in Britain and Princess Diana's struggle with the condition. The incidence rate rose dramatically in 1992, when the rumors were first published, and then again in 1994, when the speculation became rampant. It rose to its peak in 1995, when she publicly admitted the behavior. Reports of bulimia started to decline only after the princess's death in 1997. The authors consider several possible reasons for these changes. It is possible, they speculate, that Princess Di's public struggle with an eating disorder made doctors and mental health providers more aware of the condition and therefore more likely to ask about it or recognize it in their patients. They also suggest that public awareness might have made it more likely for a young woman to admit her eating behavior. Further, the apparent decline after 1997 might not indicate a true drop in the numbers, but only that fewer people weren't admitting their condition. These are reasonable hypotheses and likely explain part of the rise and fall in the numbers of bulimics. What is remarkable is that the authors of the study don't even mention, much less consider, the obvious fourth possibility: that the revelation that Princess Di used bulimia as a "call for help" *encouraged* other young women to unconsciously mimic the behavior of this beloved celebrity to call attention to their own private distress.

The fact that these researchers didn't address this possibility is emblematic of a pervasive mistaken assumption in the mental health profession: that mental illnesses exist apart from and unaffected by professional and public beliefs and the cultural currents of the time.

Off the podium, some eating disorder experts will admit to a deep insecurity about the possibility that their work might be to some degree counterproductive. I asked Michael Levine, a prominent researcher and eating disorder educator, whether he ever worries that his work has potentially spread the very disease he hopes to eradicate. "In dark periods I worry about it," he told me. "This disorder has given me an identity as a professional. I'm a tenured professor with an endowed chair. Now, am I helping people or hurting people? I hope I'm helping. But at the same time I have to acknowledge that anorexia has given me an identity in the same way it has given one to so many young girls—sometimes a deadly one."

The fact that we have not taken full account of how the professional discourse on eating disorders keeps these behaviors in the symptom pool is problematic on a number of levels. As evidenced in Hong Kong, we are engaged in globalizing our understanding, treatments, and categories of mental illness. As of now there is no acknowledgment that in doing this we may be changing the symptom pools by which people in other cultures find expression for their distress.

What does it take for a symptom such as self-starvation to exit the symptom pool? Looking back at the history of hysteria may be instructive. It was in the early part of the twentieth century that many of the symptoms of hysteria began to disappear. Hysterical fits and seizures became less common. Women in large numbers stopped reporting leg paralysis and temporary blindness and stopped collapsing while trying to walk across a room. They had fewer facial tics and involuntary muscle spasms in the arms and legs. These symptoms didn't disappear all at once, of course, but over years. During hysteria's declining years many of the symptoms seemed, at first, to lose their vigor, becoming a kind of pale version of their former selves. In France they called this *la petite hysterie*. One French doctor described women "who content themselves with a few gesticulatory movements, with a few spasms . . . and the like." So familiar were the patient and the doctor with the meaning of hysteric symptoms that little effort was required to demonstrate them. It is easy to imagine that once this milder expression of hysteria became common, it began to lose its power to communicate deep internal distress.

It may have been the very popularity of hysteria that was critical in its downfall. If part of the unconscious motivation for the hysteric was to alert the world to her internal distress, the symptoms of hysteria would lose power as they became ubiquitous. "Hysteria during the European fin de siecle came to mean so many different things that by around 1900 it ceased to mean anything at all," Mark Micale writes in his authoritative book *Approaching Hysteria: Disease and Its Interpretations*. The disease was suffering from "extreme clinical overextension." By 1930 or so, these dramatic and unmistakable symptoms began to disappear from the medical and cultural landscape as they failed to signal the distress in the unconscious minds of a new generation of women.

The decline of eating disorders may require a similar diffusion of the meaning we give them. That is to say, if anorexia and bulimia lose their ability to effectively communicate interior distress with a meaningful level of specificity, they will cease, at least for a time, to be attractive to the unconscious mind.

Looking back at the history of anorexia, it seems likely that it will someday fall back to its baseline level. But as we wait for the epidemic to subside in the West, we may have unintentionally set in motion cultural currents that will see the rise of anorexia in culture after culture around the globe.

The Lost Battle

After interviewing Ling I spent the rest of the afternoon discussing the case with Dr. Lee. He admits that she is far from cured and that his cultural sensitivity to the meaning of anorexia in Hong Kong has not led to any surefire treatments. Indeed he notes that he has lost four patients to the disease, two by starvation and two by suicide. Although his insights have not revealed a miracle cure, he believes that the only hope lies in a deep understanding of each patient's subjective experience.

At the end of our time together I asked Lee to sum up the state of the debate. He had spent the better part of two decades trying to convince the profession of psychiatry that Western assumptions about eating disorders were not only steamrolling local variations but also potentially acting as a vector, both spreading these illnesses and shaping their expression. Did he believe he had won the intellectual battle?

"No, I think the battle was lost," Lee said. "The *DSM* and Western categories for disease have gained such dominance. In the process, microcultures that shape the illness experiences of individual patients are being discarded. This is taking place around the world and not just with anorexia but with other illness categories, such as depression and ADHD [attention-deficit-hyperactivity disorder] and psychological trauma. Unfortunately the field of cross-cultural psychiatry is not doing well in terms of influencing mainstream psychiatry. I have to admit, we don't seem to interest them at all."

For a few seconds I didn't ask another question and his words hung in the air. Then Lee ended the silence. "At some point in the last ten or fifteen years the current became too strong," he said. His tone was not bitter but reflective and matter-of-fact. "It is, I think, a river of no return."

The Wave That Brought PTSD to Sri Lanka

Western mental health discourse introduces core components of Western culture, including a theory of human nature, a definition of personhood, a sense of time and memory, and a source of moral authority. None of this is universal.

DEREK SUMMERFIELD

Debra Wentz, the executive director of the New Jersey Association of Mental Health Agencies, arrived in Sri Lanka on Christmas Day 2004, one day before the tsunami that would drown more than a quarter-million people. She had traveled to the shores of the Indian Ocean for a vacation and to attend a friend's daughter's wedding. She was looking forward to a long-awaited and well-earned vacation.

She spent her first night in a cliff-side room at the Mount Lavinia Hotel just south of the capital city of Colombo. The next morning she strolled along the white sand shores below the hotel. She had planned with another wedding guest to get up early for a day trip to the historic town of Galle, a former Dutch fortress. But, tired from the previous day's travel, the pair left the hotel an hour later than they had intended. On the drive south to Galle, they stopped for a few minutes to buy some bottled water. Many lives turned on such small choices on that day.

As they were approaching Galle, a smaller wave in advance of the killer tsunami flooded the road and forced their driver to turn inland and toward higher ground. As the driver maneuvered to escape the incoming water, Wentz could see whole families running for safety. She could tell that many were in shock. "I don't think they knew they were running," she remembers. She watched helplessly as a bus struggled through the mud and rising water, unable to escape the flood. Just a few hundred yards away a train packed with travelers was swept off the tracks, killing more than eight hundred people. Wentz remembers briefly glimpsing a young woman struggling to haul an aged woman in an antiquated wheelchair away from the incoming water. The scene seemed unreal. For brief moments she felt as though she were watching an action sequence from an epic movie, something like *Gone with the Wind*. "It was like you were watching these things from outside yourself," she remembers. "I wasn't really grasping what was going on."

They were soon inland and out of sight of the water. Wentz and her companion at first had little comprehension of the magnitude of what had taken place. It was only when her driver called relatives in Galle with his cell phone that they learned that whole sections of the town had been inundated. Hundreds of people at the local bus stop had been drowned. When she finally made it back to her hotel, she took a few deep breaths to process what she had seen and consider what she could do to help. Between the rumors and news reports, she gradually became aware of the extent of the disaster. Hundreds of thousands of people had died and tens of millions had witnessed the tsunami or the death and destruction it had wrought. It was then that it dawned on her how unprepared the region was for the psychological trauma that was to come.

It was obvious to Wentz that the events of that day would have a severe, lifelong impact on the mental health of the survivors—long after their physical needs were met. As Wentz put it, "staggering acute and long-term mental health needs would remain." She had been at the helm of the New Jersey Association of Mental Health Agencies during the time of the 9/11 terrorist attacks, and from that experience she had learned a valuable lesson: the real problems with grief and post-traumatic stress disorder would come long after the event. Wentz herself could already feel the psychological effects of the tragedy she had witnessed. Her sleep became erratic and she was very emotional about the horror she had witnessed.

In the ten days she remained in the country, Wentz worked tirelessly. She moved to a hotel that had computers she could use to communicate with colleagues in the United States. Initially she focused on alerting the drug companies she worked with to the medical needs of the population. She then turned her efforts to alerting the Sri Lankan population about the devastating psychological impact that would soon be felt.

Although not a clinician herself, as head of a statewide association of 125 nonprofit behavioral health organizations, she had overseen several public service campaigns with the goal of lessening the stigma of mental illness and educating populations unaccustomed to seeking professional help. A well-connected Sri Lankan friend helped her contact the office of the prime minister. She informed an official there of the impending mental health disaster the country was facing. "I told them that this was going to be unlike anything they had experienced before," she recalls. "The psychological damage in terms of the PTSD and the anxiety and depression was only going to grow as a problem. I told them that the impact could be multigenerational."

She also contacted the Sri Lankan news media. In an interview that ran repeatedly on Sri Lankan national television in the days and weeks after the tsunami, Wentz told the population of how the symptoms of PTSD cluster in three different categories: avoidance, numbness, and hyperarousal. She advised everyone to be on the lookout for this pathological behavior in both adults and children. She told them that PTSD requires professional attention.

"I knew that the mental health needs after the tsunami would be unlike anything the world had ever seen," she recounted. "But without a sophisticated mental health system or trained counselors, where were the survivors going to turn? They had almost no psychiatrists, and most primary care doctors were not trained in psychiatry or mental health education. They didn't have a system in place to care for these people." She began to hatch a plan by which she would collect money in the United States to send American trauma experts to Sri Lanka to train local counselors how to spot and treat PTSD.

Looking back on Wentz's efforts in the hours and days after the disaster, one has to be impressed with her selflessness and genuineness of spirit. Her efforts were clearly motivated by a set of assumptions and beliefs about the nature of psychological trauma and its appropriate treatments. Wentz assumed, as do many Western mental health specialists who focus on trauma, that the psychological reaction to horrible events is fundamentally the same around the world. Had she believed otherwise, it is unlikely that she would have angled to get on Sri Lankan television to describe the coming impact of widespread PTSD. From her own recounting of the events, it is also clear that she believed that the Western world, in particular the United States, had more and better resources than the people of Sri Lanka to both understand and respond to the coming mental health crisis. Wentz's concern that Sri Lankans would have to face the psychological impact of the disaster without a "sophisticated" mental health system or "trained counselors" was repeated in many quarters during the days and months after the disaster. In every way Wentz was acting like a health professional ready to share her advanced training and knowledge to fight illness—in this case psychic wounds—in a place that lacked the knowledge and resources to care for its own.

Although Wentz was in the remarkable position of communicating directly to the Sri Lankan population in the immediate aftermath of the disaster, she was far from the only one sounding the alarm about the impending mental health epidemic. Mental health professionals around the world were telling reporters that millions of people would soon be suffering the debilitating effects of PTSD. "Traumatized Tsunami Survivors to Take Years to Heal," read the headline to a Reuters newswire story filed less than ten days after the disaster. As many as 15 to 20 percent of survivors would develop PTSD, said one expert in the Reuters story. The same expert warned that without professional counseling, as many as 16 percent of those PTSD sufferers might commit suicide. Noting that Sri Lanka already had endured much trauma from its protracted thirty-year-long civil war, Dr. Sean Scott of St. Vincent's Hospital in Sydney told a reporter from Australia's largest daily paper that the tsunami would only add to the country's psychological burden. "I believe that in the next months," Scott said, "the biggest health problem Sri Lanka and all of the region is going to be faced with is depression and post-traumatic stress disorder." Jonathan Davidson, a professor at Duke University, told a reporter, "Based on prior experience from other mass disasters, we can expect that between 50 and 90 percent of the affected population will experience conditions like post-traumatic stress disorder and depression which, if untreated, may last for years."

Although the estimated percentage of people who would be affected varied widely from expert to expert, there was a clear consensus among those experts that the need for psychological treatment services would overwhelm the available providers in the region. Those experts also generally agreed that getting to the scene quickly was critical. "Psychological scarring needs to be dealt with as quickly as possible," a psychologist told the *Washington Post* in the days after the tsunami. "The longer we wait, the more damage." The metaphor of a wave was unavoidable. Many Western reporters and experts talked about a "second tsunami" of mental illness that could be avoided only if proper support and treatment were given. Responding to the dire warnings, hundreds of nongovernmental organizations, universities, and private groups quickly began to gather resources and make plans to send an army of trauma counselors in teams of various sizes to the coastal areas of the Indian Ocean.

What happened over the next months in Sri Lanka, Indonesia, India, and Thailand was likely the largest international psychological intervention of all time. Trauma counselors and researchers poured into the region not only from the United States, but also from Britain, France, Australia, and New Zealand. As part of its billion-dollar pledge of assistance, Australia sent multiple teams of counselors with the intent to bring the mental health services in the region "into the modern era." The director of AusAID, Robin Davies, said that the effort was not intended to restore or rebuild the mental health care capacity in the country. "Restore is the wrong word," Davies was quoted as saying, "because there was nothing much there before."

Given the certainty surrounding the need for such an effort, it is remarkable to remember that we are the first generation to include psychological first aid with other forms of assistance after wars and disasters. As late as the mid-1980s, in fact, the manuals for postdisaster relief focused exclusively on medicine, food, and shelter and contained no advice for treating the psychological wounds of a population.

It's only been in the past twenty years that the diagnosis of PTSD has caught the world's attention. It first gained critical momentum in the United States and then began leapfrogging the globe, being put to use after wars, genocides, and natural disasters. By 2004 PTSD was on the cusp of becoming the international lingua franca of human suffering. We were suddenly in a time when, as one psychiatrist put it, the concern over psychological trauma had "displaced hunger as the first thing the Western general public thinks about when a war or other emergency is in the news."

"We were spreading these ideas around the globe so effectively that PTSD was becoming the way the entire world conceived of psychological trauma," said Allan Young, a medical anthropologist at McGill University who has studied the history of PTSD. "The spread of the PTSD diagnosis to every corner of the world may, in the end, be the greatest success story of globalization."

Seldom considered in our rush to help treat the psychic wounds of traumatized people was the question of whether PTSD was a diagnosis that could be usefully applied in all human cultures.

The idea that people from different cultures might have fundamentally different psychological reactions to a traumatic event is hard for Americans to grasp. The human body's visceral reaction to trauma—adrenaline, fear, and the fight-or-flight response—is so primal that we assume that the aftereffects of such events would also be the same everywhere. The symptoms that make up PTSD, which include intrusive thoughts and dreams, memory avoidance, and uncontrollable anxiety and arousal when the victim is reminded of the event,* seem utterly commonsensical.

---

*As the *DSM-IV* describes PTSD: "The essential feature of Post-traumatic Stress Disorder is the development of characteristic symptoms following exposure to an extreme traumatic stressor involving direct personal experience of an event that involves actual or threatened death or serious injury, or other threat to one's physical integrity; or witnessing an event that involves death, injury, or a threat to the physical integrity of another person; or learning about unexpected or violent death, serious harm, or threat of death or injury experienced by a family member or other close associate (Criterion A1). The person's response to

But PTSD isn't just a list of symptoms. Since PTSD was added to the *DSM* in 1980, Western mental health researchers and clinicians have devoted vast amounts of time and energy researching and treating psychological trauma. Indeed if you were an ambitious researcher in psychology or psychiatry during the 1990s, PTSD was where the action was; by 2004 more than twenty thousand articles, books, and reports had been indexed in the National Center for Post-Traumatic Stress Disorder's database. Just as hysteria was the archetypal disorder of the Victorian era, PTSD speaks volumes about how Americans and the Western world conceive of the self.

Those mental health professionals who formed our generation's understanding of PTSD have created an intricate labyrinth of ideas that includes explicit and implicit assumptions about what type of event will damage the human mind and who will be most affected. Within the literature of this movement are prescriptions for how, as individuals and as a society, we should react to horrible events and what types of resources we should devote to the victims. Farther back in this labyrinth of meaning one encounters still other ideas: calls for solidarity with the survivors of violence; incitements to share an enlightened moral outrage against the atrocities of war and social injustice; the belief that the study of PTSD has made us more attuned and sensitive to the world's suf-

---

the event must involve intense fear, helplessness, or horror (or in children, the response must involve disorganized or agitated behavior) (Criterion A2). The characteristic symptoms resulting from the exposure to the extreme trauma include persistent reexperiencing of the traumatic event (Criterion B), persistent avoidance of stimuli associated with the trauma and numbing of general responsiveness (Criterion C), and persistent symptoms of increased arousal (Criterion D). The full symptom picture must be present for more than 1 month (Criterion E), and the disturbance must cause clinically significant distress or impairment in social, occupational, or other important areas of functioning (Criterion F)."

fering. Taken as a whole, this body of knowledge goes far beyond describing a disorder with a symptom cluster. It describes a worldview.

Western traumatologists have also developed a set of beliefs about how best to heal from the psychological effects of trauma. They have proposed that speedy interventions to counsel survivors within hours or days of the event are crucial; that retelling or reworking the memories of the trauma, often in emotionally charged group settings, promotes mental health; and that truth telling is better for the mind than stoic silence. Against a growing body of evidence, traumatologists assume these ideas to be universally true.

Traumatologists have also advanced the idea that psychological rehabilitation is best managed by mental health experts, certified in and sensitized to the Western understanding of how humans suffer and heal. The post-tsunami intervention would prove to be a crucible for these Western certainties.

Kate Chaos

One of the traumatologists who heard the call to help those suffering in Sri Lanka was Kate Amatruda, a therapist from northern California. Just days after the tsunami she found a message in her email in-box from the Association for Play Therapy seeking volunteers for an urgent mission to the disaster zone. She immediately faxed her application and was selected to be part of a team of a dozen play therapists who would be dispatched to help children suffering mental trauma in orphanages and local community centers. She was expected to be on a plane within ten days.

Among the many letters representing her credentials (MFT,

CST-T, DMAT, DSHR-DMH) Amatruda is a BCETS, a Board Certified Expert in Traumatic Stress. Seen in a broader context, she is one of thousands of American therapists and mental health professionals who, in the past twenty-five years, tied their careers to the remarkable ascendancy of PTSD in American psychiatry and public consciousness. Amatruda had become well known in the field. She regularly gave speeches and taught courses on the subject at local universities and online, training young therapists to recognize PTSD. She also taught the techniques for how best to heal from the disorder, usually through a nondirective approach based on retelling, playing, and drawing. Amatruda was traveling to Sri Lanka to apply her knowledge where it was needed most.

Amatruda is a short woman with bubbly energy and a mane of long, curly, graying blond hair. She self-effacingly admits that her family often calls her "Kate Chaos," a reference to her often frenzied state. In the week before her departure, she worked frantically to put her professional and personal life on hold. Preparing for her mission, she bought mosquito repellant, antacids, antidiarrhea pills, Advil, anti-itch cream, Wet Wipes, toilet paper, and hand sanitizer—enough supplies, she wrote, to "feel like a walking pharmacy." She also collected donations of art supplies from several schools in her town. In one large suitcase she packed sixty-nine pounds of balloons, scissors, paper and paper punches, pens, glue, stickers, and "zillions" of children's Band-Aids. Through bake sales she also raised two hundred dollars that she planned to take with her and donate to a worthy local group.

From my examination of her extensive writing on the subject, I think Amatruda sees trauma as forming a kind of psychic infection in the mind and the best way to drain that infection is through retelling the story. The purpose of play and art therapy is to open nonverbal ways of mastering the traumatic memory.

Such techniques, which emphasize retelling or reworking the trauma verbally or otherwise in the days immediately after a horror, are in the tradition of what has been called "psychological first aid," or sometimes "critical incident debriefing." The basic idea, developed and promoted in the United States throughout the 1990s, is that the earlier a victim begins to "process" or "master" the memory of the trauma, the less likely that memory will form the kind of mental abscess that results in PTSD. Counselors clearly see themselves as akin to emergency medical professionals treating wounds at the scene of the accident. Their charge is to deliver the psychological equivalent of applying clean dressings to fresh wounds.

In this way of thinking, it hardly seemed to matter that most of the trauma counselors headed to Sri Lanka had little understanding of the culture they were entering. Few could comprehend the local languages, nor were they experts on the population's religious beliefs, its grieving and burial rituals, or the country's long and complicated history of civil war.

But such a lack of knowledge was no deterrent to administering aid. In her writing, Amatruda states emphatically, "One of the requirements of disaster response is to be non-political, non-denominational, and nondiscriminatory. . . . We offer aid by need, not religion, ethnicity, political affiliation, etc." If you're doing the mental health equivalent of applying a compress to someone's injured head, why would you need to share his or her religious beliefs, traditions, or social structures?

Clearly in Denial

The assumption that traumatic reactions exist outside and unaffected by culture was common among both individual trauma counselors and the relief organizations sponsoring them. Dr. Sebastian von Peter, from the Hospital of Neukölln in Berlin, took the time to read through all the advisory texts and manuals related to the treatment of trauma after the tsunami. Mostly written by teams of international mental health experts to help train relief workers and volunteers, these texts were produced by CARE, the Red Cross International, the World Health Organization (WHO), the Global Development Group, the National Center for Post-Traumatic Stress Disorder, and the European Society for Traumatic Event Studies, among others. These organizations and agencies, he wrote, assume that "at root, people throughout the world are the same in their emotional experience and expressions." Taken together, von Peter concluded, these manuals imply a universal metaphysic of emotional experience. In the face of horror, these manuals assume, all humans are fundamentally the same.

Despite these certainties, there were signs early on after the tsunami of a cultural disconnect between the ideas surrounding the Western conception of PTSD and Sri Lankan beliefs. There was, for instance, a remarkable memo emailed just days after the disaster by faculty members from the University of Colombo in Sri Lanka. The professors acknowledged that "disaster zones attract 'trauma' and 'counseling projects,'" but they pleaded with the arriving army of counselors not to reduce survivors' experiences "to a question of mental trauma" and the survivors themselves to "psychological casualties."

They went on to make an argument that fundamentally undercut the certainty that Western ideas about trauma are universal. "A victim processes a traumatic event as a function of what it means," they wrote. "This meaning is drawn from their society and culture and this shapes how they seek help and their expectation of recovery." Trauma reactions aren't automatic physiological reactions inside the brain, they suggested, but rather cultural communications. They have nuance and meaning that can be misinterpreted or overlooked unless observers have a deep understanding of the culture at hand. What was required before any organization could offer meaningful help, the professors wrote, was a deep understanding of "what the affected people were signaling by this distress."

In the days after the disaster, reporters and clinicians arriving from the United States and elsewhere sometimes seemed confused, even concerned, when the local population didn't behave the way they'd expected. One trauma counselor being interviewed on BBC radio from a small coastal village expressed his worry that the local children appeared more interested in returning to school than discussing their experience of the tsunami. These children were "clearly in denial," the expert told the listening audience. The host of the program concurred, saying, "Of course, everyone knows that children are the most vulnerable to trauma such as this." The expert then confidently concluded that only later would the children "experience the full emotional horror of what has happened to them." Similarly CNN reporters expressed their amazement when tens of thousands of Sri Lankans attempted to abandon their refugee camps just days after the disaster, preferring to go back to their devastated villages or depend on friends or family. A *New York Times* reporter wrote that it would be only "a matter of time" before the "wall of determination and denial, which has enabled so many to cope in the days immediately after the Dec. 26 tsunami disaster, begins to break down."

With so many counseling and trauma treatment programs and PTSD researchers arriving in the country every day, the situation on the ground soon turned chaotic. Shekhar Saxena, from the World Health Organization, was disturbed by the scene he saw in the days and weeks after the tsunami. "Two weeks after the tsunami there were hundreds of counselors doing nothing or getting in the way," he told a reporter from Reuters. He pointed out that sending mental health workers who didn't speak the local language or understand the culture was as useless as sending the wrong medicines.

Dr. Mahesan Ganesan, who was the only psychiatrist in all of eastern Sri Lanka, desperately tried to keep track of the various organizations arriving to give psychological aid. For a few days he managed to keep a tally of the dozens of groups on a large whiteboard in his office, but he soon lost count.

Looking back, it's hard to escape the feeling that these various efforts had about them the energy and excitement of a gold rush. The tsunami was one of the most devastating natural disasters in recorded history, and everyone who wanted to demonstrate their acumen in healing trauma or perform large-scale studies of PTSD felt obligated to be on the scene. If a technique was to be taken seriously as a treatment for psychological trauma, its adherents had to be part of the action.

Within days bitter rivalries broke out between counseling groups over which populations would receive which services. As one journalist documented, different support services attempted to "stake their claim to refugee camps." The haggling between groups vying to help sometimes caused confusion and bad feelings among the survivors. One Sri Lankan health care worker described how children were lured away from one set of volunteer mental health care providers by other groups with toys and other incentives. "Children are torn between these loyalties, and it can be traumatic," said T. Gadambanathan, a Sri Lankan psychiatrist from Trincomalee.

Similarly Ganesan watched with a mixture of horror and fascination as several organizations offering counseling services to one camp fought among themselves for the attention of the children. "It was common for the [facilitators] to differentiate between 'our' children and 'their' children," he reports. "At times children were asked not to play with children belonging to other groups. This often led to conflicts . . . and at times brought about animosity between the children themselves."

Ganesan noted a key difference between the aid groups offering medicine, food, and shelter and those offering trauma counseling. The groups focusing on basic material needs would immediately meet with local officials and families to try to assess what the community was lacking. Was shelter the first priority, or food, or first aid? In contrast, those setting up PTSD counseling services seldom asked leaders in the local community what they needed or desired in terms of help. Thinking back, Ganesan's considered several possible reasons for this lack of consultation. Perhaps these traumatologists felt that the local community did not understand their own psychological needs, and therefore "getting their opinion would be a pointless waste of time." More likely, he's concluded, these trauma counselors shared the "idea that all persons would respond in a psychologically known manner to trauma and loss, and a particular universal method existed to help these people whoever they were and whatever their culture." Such a belief would make consultation with the local population unnecessary.

There were other problems. Translators had to be employed, as nearly none of the trauma counselors arriving from Western countries spoke the local languages. Given all the foreign activity in the country, the most proficient translators were in high demand. This meant that counselors often relied on those with marginal translation skills, such as local drivers who plied the tourist trade, to facilitate their therapy sessions. "At best [these translators] had very limited capacity to translate the very complicated and sensitive communication that takes place during a counseling session," noted one local health worker.

Despite such difficulties, the pace of counseling often rivaled the speed of an emergency room. Over two four-day periods in late

January and February, one organization reported giving "psycho-therapy and counseling" to 1,724 people, including 631 children. This was an impressive feat given that they had only two dozen counselors to do the work. Another group of Western counselors debriefed twenty-five traumatized survivors at a time, with the goal of one hundred treated for each five hours of work.

The drug company Pfizer was quick to get in the mix as well. In early February 2005, just over a month after the disaster, the company sponsored a symposium in Bangkok titled "After the Tsunami: Mental Health Challenges to the Community for Today and Tomorrow." Professor Davidson, quoted earlier predicting pathology rates of 50 to 90 percent, helped organize the conference with an "unrestricted grant" from the company.

The paper Davidson presented at the conference was titled "Pharmacologic Treatment of Acute and Chronic Stress Following Trauma." He described PTSD as "a severe, chronic, and disabling condition with major consequences for the individual and society," but assured his audience that antidepressants such as Pfizer's Zoloft could become "an effective tool in promoting the long-term psychological and psychosocial health, and economic recovery, of those in the region affected by the tsunami." Zoloft, he reported, had been shown to reduce anger after the first week of treatment and lessen "emotional upset" by week six. By the tenth week of treatment, those who took the drug were less likely to avoid trauma-related activities. Although Zoloft had been approved for PTSD only a few years prior, Davidson described the drug treatment as "currently recommended as first-line therapy for the treatment of PTSD" in the United States.

According to World Health Organization observers, fewer than half of the trauma counseling groups that flooded the country bothered to register with the government. Fewer still worked to coordinate their efforts with each other. "There was no checking," John Mahoney, the director of the World Health Organization's mental health initiative in Sri Lanka, told a reporter. "We found one organization just handing out anti-depressants to people."

A People's Army of Trauma Therapists

In addition to the assembly-line counseling, Western experts on the ground in Sri Lanka took to training the locals in the latest techniques of treating PTSD. Sri Lankans, generally speaking, have an intense hunger and respect for education. That these Westerners, with their impressive credentials, would be offering free training in modern healing methods seemed a stroke of good fortune. Thousands of Sri Lankans took advantage of the offer, packing the training sessions, which were sometimes as long as two weeks but often as brief as a day.

A team of educators from the University of Pennsylvania and Swarthmore traveled to the region to train one hundred master teachers in a child-centered brand of educational psychology that uses the creation of illustrated storybooks to give survivors a method to retell their stories. A group of American therapists and social workers calling itself the Heart Circle Sangha also arrived to "train Sri Lankan counselors and leave in Sri Lanka a cadre of skilled clinicians" who would have "techniques for working with intense grief and Post-traumatic Stress Disorder." According to their literature, the group taught "skills of deep listening, empathy, the healing power of connection. . . . The project emphasizes counseling skills that empower clients." The Humanitarian Committee of the Association for Comprehensive Energy Psychology, sometimes called thought field therapy, sent counselors to Sri Lanka to provide free treatment and training for the local population. These energy psychologists tapped on parts of the body while encouraging the patient to bring up anxious thoughts and traumatic memories. Practitioners of eye movement desensitization and reprocessing (EMDR) also offered training sessions to locals. In EMDR, which is supposed to resolve symptoms of PTSD, the therapist instructs patients to follow a moving object from side to side with their eyes while holding a mental picture of the disturbing life event in their mind.

The Western experts leading these sessions often reported frustration at having to school their trainees in the most basic concepts of Western therapy. Mary Cattan, who was part of another training effort in Sri Lanka, found the locals eager but psychologically unsophisticated. They were so interested in giving practical advice, she recounts, that "their listening skills were not very good." More problematic still was the fact that the local trainees were "not particularly self-aware."

Usually, everyone was invited to attend these trainings, including children. "After a while, most youngsters in Batticaloa had acquired certificates which indicated that they had received training in counseling," noted one Sri Lankan observer.

The effectiveness of this new people's army of trauma counselors concerned some. There simply wasn't enough time or resources to provide supervision for these newly minted counselors or to put in place safeguards should they run into difficult or dangerous clinical situations. Asked about these issues, the foreign trainers would wave off the concern by assuring the questioner that they weren't, in fact, training "counselors." Rather, they said, these were "befrienders" or "community support officers," as if the renaming solved the inherent problem. It's clear, however, that these freshly trained locals often believed that they were now armed with Western-tested knowledge about how to treat those in distress.

Mixed in among the therapists and counselors was another large contingent of Western PTSD specialists: the trauma researchers. Like the counselors, those who specialized in the scientific study of psychological trauma couldn't afford to miss this once-in-a-lifetime disaster. One of the first research groups on the scene, from the University of Konstanz in Germany, looked for posttraumatic stress disorder among children in Sri Lanka starting just three weeks after the disaster. Studying several locations, they soon reported finding PTSD rates between 14 and 39 percent.*

Some of the researchers employed cutting-edge technology. One team went to various refugee camps shortly after the disaster collecting blood samples to measure chemicals indicative of stress reactions. Another group of researchers used a polygraph machine to record heart rate, breathing, and skin resistance. Researchers interested in genetic predispositions for PTSD were particularly keen about the opportunity the tsunami presented. They noted that because whole families were simultaneously exposed to the tsunami, the event provided a unique opportunity to look at subtle differences in genes that would lead one family member to develop PTSD and another family member to psychologically recover in short order. In one multimillion-dollar study three thousand tsunami survivors were interviewed and more than six hundred sufferers of PTSD identified. Researchers then drew blood from those afflicted as well as their healthy siblings in hopes of finding gene sequences to explain their differing psychological reactions.

From the perspective of the locals, there was a good deal of confusion regarding the trauma researchers, who were suddenly swarming refugee camps asking deeply personal questions, requesting

---

*For some critics, this very first study became emblematic of the rush to diagnose PTSD. How could PTSD have been diagnosed starting at three weeks, some wondered, when the definition of the disorder requires the symptoms to last for longer than one month?

samples of their blood, and sometimes hooking them up to strange machines. To begin with, the distinction between those who came to treat them and those who came primarily to study them was often unclear. The researchers appeared to be just one more tent of concerned foreigners set up on the periphery of a refugee camp.

In a report to the Sri Lankan Parliament, Dr. Athula Sumathipala pointed out the ethical problems inherent in such a situation: "When research is combined with aid, relief and at times clinical care, there is undue inducement for participation in this vulnerable population." Because Sri Lanka lacked any comprehensive process to review and approve research involving humans, the country was being invaded by what he called "parachute researchers."

Sumathipala pointed out that many Sri Lankans who had never participated in a research study before didn't fully understand that they had the choice not to answer the questions of the investigators. More disturbing still, locals sometimes assumed their participation would lead to some financial assistance or other help. From the perspective of the victims, it made sense that those gathering such detailed information about their hardships would be connected to some form of assistance down the road. Why else would they be so interested?

One American observer, who asked to remain anonymous, sat in on a seminar held by a large international nongovernmental organization that promised to train teachers how to counsel children with posttraumatic stress disorder. In reality, the actual focus of the two-day session was to show the teachers how to complete a PTSD symptom checklist. Although attendees thought they were learning new skills in dealing with traumatized children, they were actually being trained in data collection for a study of the prevalence of PTSD. Within weeks of the tsunami these trainees were sent into classrooms to collect data not only on the children's reactions to the trauma but also on their history of domestic violence and sexual abuse.

Further blurring the line between research and assistance was the fact that dozens of the studies were designed to assess the validity of one treatment or another. Which is to say that groups of locals were encouraged to participate in some style of experimental counseling or therapy for the purposes of determining that treatment's efficacy. One research group, for instance, conducted a study in which they organized groups of adult and child tsunami survivors to revisit the exact locations where they experienced the disaster. The idea was that reexposing them to the scenes where they witnessed the disaster would help them process the experience. Afterward the study's authors reported somewhat cryptically, "No certain cases of retraumatization occurred [among the participants]." Nowhere did they make clear whether the participants understood there was such a risk.

Most of the studies conducted in the weeks and months after the tsunami were of a simple nature. With local assistance, Western researchers translated up-to-date PTSD questionnaires and employed them to assess the mental health of a given population. These surveys were designed mostly by researchers in the United States to quickly determine—usually with fewer than two dozen questions—if the symptoms of PTSD were present. Children in Phuket and Krabi, Thailand, were studied with the UCLA PTSD Reaction; children in the Ranong province of Thailand and others in Tangalle in the southern province of Sri Lanka were assessed with the Children's Impact Events Scale 13, which is referred to among trauma specialists as the CRIES-13. The population of northern Sumatra and Aceh, Indonesia, were assessed using the Post-traumatic Stress Disorder Checklist–Civilian Version. Adults in Tamil Nadu, India, were given the Harvard Trauma Questionnaire. The resulting studies published in peer-reviewed journals universally reported significant rates of PTSD among the cohorts studied.

For many trauma researchers, these results unambiguously settle the question of whether PTSD was present after the tsunami. But there is a more difficult and telling question here: Did the information gathered from those PTSD surveys accurately represent the distress being experienced by these populations?

"When you ask [the] whole checklist, the classical PTSD criteria would be there, but these are all leading questions," one Sri Lankan medical specialist was quoted as observing. "When you ask 'do you have intrusive memories?'. . . It is easier to say 'intrusive memory' in English, but [try] to put it into Sinhala or Tamil. You see, is very difficult and by the time you have explained all that, they know that they have to answer in the positive."

The very act of asking survivors to describe their psychological response to a horrible experience by choosing among only a few reactions would seem to unavoidably bias the outcome. Adding to this problem was the common misperception on the part of those being studied that answering such questions "correctly" would result in assistance for oneself or one's family.

Further complicating matters was an implicit assumption imbedded in these PTSD checklists: that the traumatic event in question was a one-off experience safely in the past and that life had otherwise gone back to normal. It might indeed be pathological to be constantly on the watch for danger six months after an anomalous event, such as witnessing a violent crime. But for those living with their children in the squalor and discord of a refugee camp, being vigilant about safety would certainly have a different meaning. Unfortunately it was impossible for any of the PTSD surveys to make a meaningful distinction between the psychological reaction to the tsunami and the ongoing strains of the social and economic turmoil caused by that event.

In the end these trauma checklists simply had no ability to discover what might be culturally unique to the experience of living through horror in Sri Lanka. These surveys weren't designed to discover anything new, but rather to confirm similarities. Did the population have other reactions to the trauma not included in the symptom lists? Were the behaviors on the checklists the reactions that caused the most concern to the Sri Lankans? Such questions didn't seem to occur to the researchers, who appeared to believe wholeheartedly in the universality of the PTSD construct.

Resilience in Sri Lanka

Dr. Gaithri Fernando, a young assistant professor of psychology at California State University in Los Angeles, was with her son in Sri Lanka on high ground when the tsunami of 2004 rolled ashore. In a bizarre coincidence, she was in the region preparing a study on the psychological impact of a 2001 earthquake. After the wave receded, she traveled to the fishing village of Moratuwa, where she saw people frozen in disbelief and horror. It was clear that the wave had inflicted both psychological and physical damage.

Fernando watched with increasing unease as scores of Western psychologists, counselors, and PTSD researchers arrived in the disaster zone. A native of Sri Lanka, and a mix of Tamil and Sinhalese, Fernando moved to the United States when she was 21 to help her husband, a Tamil, escape persecution. Since then she has returned often to conduct research on the psychological impact of the long civil war. The wave of aid that rolled in on Sri Lanka after the tsunami, she suspected, had the power to change the culture of the island country as much as the tsunami itself.

Few understand better than Fernando the Sri Lankan capacity to live in the face of horror. Her research prior to the tsunami documents a people with remarkable psychological resilience. Even through decades of war, youth uprisings, and poverty, most Sri Lankans have managed to remain functional and hopeful. This is a population, she has shown, that seldom needed outside encouragement or counseling to get back on its feet even after the most punishing hardships.

Many of the Western counselors and experts who rushed in after the tsunami assumed that the long and brutal civil war had made the individuals in the population ever more psychologically vulnerable and therefore more likely to experience PTSD after the tsunami. There was, of course, an alternative possibility: that the Sri Lankans—*because of their intimate familiarity with poverty, hardship, and war*—had evolved a culture better able to integrate and give meaning to terrible events. In this conception it was the Western counselors, arriving from communities and enclaves unfamiliar with the immediate experience of violence and deprivation, who were uniquely vulnerable.

Fernando knows how Sri Lankans turn to their rich cultural traditions in times of hardship. Religion is a particularly important cornerstone in the lives of most. There are Buddhist traditions for the majority Sinhalese, Hinduism for the Tamils, Islam for the Moors, and Christianity for the rest. The notion of karma, central to both Buddhist and Hindu beliefs, is shared by Sri Lankans across ethnic and religious lines. Overlapping and weaving together these different traditions is the shared ethnocultural belief in spirits and the palpable nearness of the spirit world.

Often closely tied to religious traditions is a wide variety of healing customs. Health care in Sri Lanka is remarkably pluralistic. There are Ayurvedic practitioners, doctors, astrologers, religious leaders, mediums, and faith healers of various types. The lines between these practices, delineating, for instance, traditional healing from modern medicine, are not clearly drawn. A Sri Lankan often consults two or more of these traditions in search of relief from illness or psychological distress.

Having watched at close quarters the suffering of children and their parents caught in the violence of the civil war, Fernando intimately understands that these cultural traditions have an impact not only on the ways this population talks about the psychological aftermath of horror but on the deeper level of how it is felt and experienced. She understands, as those Colombo professors said immediately after the tsunami, that victims process traumatic events as a product of what they mean.

Indeed Fernando's earlier work on war trauma in Sri Lanka had uncovered fascinating connections between religious beliefs and differences in the ability to recover from the trauma of war. In one pre-tsunami study she found that Buddhist and Hindu children who experienced war and violence were less vulnerable to depression than Christian children, even though the Buddhist and Hindu kids reported more personal exposure, witnessing bomb blasts and the like. She speculated that there might be protective beliefs in Hindu and Buddhist traditions, such as the active acceptance of pain and suffering or the beliefs in rebirth and recompense through reincarnation, that steadied these children in the wake of terror.

Watching the aftermath of the tsunami, Fernando couldn't, of course, predict the psychological consequences. This was an unprecedented event that could overtax the religious institutions and healing traditions that the population relied on. Still, the idea, often repeated by Western experts, that Sri Lankans had few local resources for psychological healing (because they lacked trauma counselors) seemed to simply ignore or discount the cultural traditions, beliefs, and rituals that Sri Lankans had so long relied on. Similarly the idea common to many Western traumatologists, that psychological treatments could be easily divorced from religion, ethnicity, and the cultural history of the country, was hard for Fernando to understand.

Most important, Fernando worried that the PTSD symptom

checklists did not reflect the culturally particular ways that Sri Lankans experience psychological suffering after trauma. She worried that by using these checklists mental health professionals from Western countries would be ineffective—or even do harm—unless they understood that Sri Lankans had culturally distinct reactions to traumatic events as well as culturally specific modes of healing. She believed that unless these local idioms of distress were understood, appropriate interventions could not be formulated. Without a deep understanding of the illness, in other words, it would be impossible to treat the disease.

Fernando took on the task of trying to understand the local meaning of trauma in post-tsunami Sri Lanka. She began by gathering a sample of local informants from a rural area in the southern province of the country. All were Sinhalese Buddhists, most from poor families. All had personally witnessed the tsunami, and fifteen of the twenty had lost family members.

Instead of quizzing these subjects with a predetermined set of PTSD symptoms, Fernando asked each person to tell her two open-ended stories in their own language. First she asked participants to think of someone they knew who had experienced some type of suffering but was now functioning well. After that story was finished, the subject was asked to describe a person who was functioning poorly after a traumatic event.

Not surprisingly, of the forty stories she collected, thirty-five were related to the tsunami. With the help of a researcher and a local community leader, she began to examine the narratives for similarities in themes and expressions of wellness and distress. In the end she collected more than two dozen symptoms and behaviors that were mentioned by fifteen or more participants. She then validated the results by conducting a large-scale survey. She ended up with what she calls the Sri Lankan Index of Psychosocial Status, a twenty-six-item measure of the local indicators of distress.

Fernando came to the conclusion that Sri Lankans' experience of trauma differed from Americans' in two main ways. Unlike the PTSD symptomatology, Sri Lankans were much more likely to experience physical symptoms after horrible events. Sri Lankans who lost family members or whose lives were otherwise devastated by the tsunami were more likely to complain of aches in the joints or muscles or pain in the chest. Without the mind-body disconnect common in Western thinking, these Sri Lankans reacted to the disaster as if they had experienced a physical blow to the body.

In addition to these somatic symptoms, there was another, more subtle and pervasive difference. By and large Sri Lankans didn't report pathological reactions to trauma in line with the internal states (anxiety, fear, numbing, and the like) that make up most of the PTSD symptom checklist. Rather Sri Lankans tended to see the negative consequences of an event like the tsunami in terms of the damage it did to social relationships. Those who continued to suffer long after a horrible experience, her research showed, were those who had become isolated from their social network or who were not fulfilling their role in kinship groups. In short, they conceived of the damage done by the tsunami as occurring not inside their mind but outside the self, in the social environment.

Such social problems are also common in Western sufferers of PTSD, but Fernando's research highlighted a subtle but important distinction. In Western thinking surrounding PTSD a trauma causes psychological damage that then results in social problems. A Westerner might, for instance, assume that depression or anxiety brought on by PTSD would cause people to fail in their role as a parent. For a Sri Lankan, this did not appear to be a cause-and-effect phenomenon. The failure to manage one's social responsibilities—to find and fulfill a place in the group—was identified as the primary symptom of distress and not a consequence of an internal psychological problem. As she concluded in her paper on the subject, "The data empirically support the theory that intra-psychic functioning is not independent from interpersonal functioning for this community." On examination of the interviews, Fernando realized that every one of the twenty-six symptoms described by these Sri Lankans was to some extent bound to this idea that the social trumped the psychological. More precisely, Sri Lankans interwove the social and the psychological—to the point where the two could not be teased apart. Because the Western conception of PTSD assumes the problem, the breakage, is primarily in the mind of the individual, it largely overlooks the most salient symptoms for a Sri Lankan, those that exist not in the psychological but in the social realm.

This is one of those subtle cultural differences that is hard to point to at any given time. In trying to describe the interconnection between the social and the individual sense of well-being, Fernando told me of interviewing a young boy in a village that had been the scene of several massacres. The boy was 8 years old, and his father had been killed during one of the periods of violence. Fernando was working with another researcher who didn't speak the local language, and so she was translating the questions and answers so the other professor could understand. At one point she asked the boy what makes him feel better when he gets worried about the violence in his community, and the boy answered that it was the things his mother says to him. "This boy told me that he feels better when his mother promises him that if they are attacked and killed that they would all die together," Fernando recalls. The answer struck her so deeply that for several moments she couldn't translate the response for the other researcher. The mother offered no promise of protection or even survival, only togetherness in the face of violence and death. The boy, for his part, appeared deeply reassured by his mother's promise.

This emphasis on the social over the psychological becomes critical when one considers how one might heal from tragic events. If depression, anxiety, or hypervigilance are the primary symptoms (which then lead to social problems in one's family or social group), it might make sense to take time to work though the psychological symptoms away from one's social responsibilities. This is a common pattern of mental health healing in the West: take a sick leave from the stresses in your life in order to heal. If, however, the social difficulties are the primary symptom of distress, taking time away from one's duties and social roles to pursue something like individual counseling may actually exacerbate the problem. In a culture such as Sri Lanka's, an emphasis on healing the individual away from the group, particularly in one-on-one counseling with strangers, is problematic.

A Guide to Post-Traumatic Fieldwork

Based on her experiences in Sri Lanka and subsequently in New Orleans after Hurricane Katrina, Kate Amatruda has written "A Field Guide to Disaster Mental Health," which comes as part of an online course that is sold on the Internet for $110, and is approved for continuing education by organizations including the Association for Play Therapy and the National Association of Social Workers. It's a perplexing document, part journal of her adventures, part how-to guide for those hoping to work in disaster zones.

In her field guide, Amatruda assures the reader of how culturally sensitive she remained. She reports that, on arrival, she was given a full day's training in Sri Lankan customs and history. Local officials instructed her to wear her hair up and to eat only with her right hand. She was also told that she couldn't ask children to play a card game called Go Fish because the "fish aspect" could be a "trauma trigger"; in addition, she was told that all card games or other activities that might be construed as gambling were forbidden among Muslims.

On a personal level, she reports in her online "Tsunami Journal" having experienced some culture shock on her arrival. The normal discomforts of traveling in a developing nation were heightened in the aftermath of the disaster. The lack of showers and Western-style toilets also took some getting used to, and the curry dishes she ate for breakfast didn't agree with her stomach. She remembers being constantly anxious about contracting head lice from the children in the camps. She describes being particularly pleased with the training sessions she helped conduct with local teachers and health care workers.

In reviewing the field guide, I found it difficult to discern what particular practices Amatruda brought to Sri Lanka. The guide recommends encouraging "the children to express their feelings" and that helpers should listen "without passing judgment." It also cautions against a "rush back to ordinary school routines too soon," because children and adolescents should have "time to talk over the traumatic event and expresss their feelings about it." She writes of leading dances and songs with the children and that her team performed cognitive behavior puppet shows and games "geared toward the mastery of trauma." She also reports using "mirror neurons" to establish a deep connection with those she counseled.

"In disaster work," she writes, "it helps to match body language, tone, volume, and eye contact of the host culture . . . [this is] particularly important when people are extremely stressed, and when there are cultural differences. We want to impart on a non-verbal basis that we are here for you, we are not a threat, and we are trying, at the most basic level of our consciousness, the cellular, to show up and empathize."

But even though she repeatedly talks of the need to "train the trainers," exactly what information, techniques, or processes were taught—and why those were selected above all other interventions—is left vague.

Many counselors returning from their work in Sri Lanka were loath to be seen as part of some hegemonic West-to-East, rich-to-poor transfer of knowledge. Recounting their counseling and training work after the tsunami, some Western traumatologists went to almost comic extremes to assure their readers or questioners that they were sensitive to the local culture. Dr. John R. Van Eenwyk, the founder and clinical director of the International Trauma Treatment Program, curiously insisted that the best role for Western trauma trainers was to prove that they had nothing to offer their trainees. The intent of the trainings he conducted in Sri Lanka was to reveal himself to be as powerless as the Wizard of Oz. "Our job is to reveal ourselves as 'the man behind the curtain,'" he explained. "Then we help them see that what they seek from us they already possess. Like the scarecrow, they already have brains. . . . We don't indoctrinate. We empower."

Despite these demurrals, one is often struck in these retellings that it is the Western healer who takes center stage. A significant amount of Amatruda's field guide, for instance, is devoted to documenting how deeply she and her fellow counselors experienced the events. When seeing the destruction at the beach she writes: "We are shocked, speechless, horrified. There are no words. . . . We are stunned into silence." At the orphanage, she reports, "my heart breaks again and again and again. . . . Daily debriefing became very important to us, as we needed to help each other deal with the torrent of loss and pain we were facing and feeling. The name for this phenomenon is 'vicarious traumatization'; it describes how a person can feel holding so much of another's pain." One begins to suspect that this type of hyper-empathy (in the field guide, counselors are described as having "extrasensory radar") is actually the gift these healers believe they are delivering.

In her online journal, Amatruda tells how one day, not long after her arrival, she was counseling a woman named Selvie-amah, who was the housemother for an orphanage of girls. When Selvie-amah revealed that she had lost two brothers in the civil war, Amatruda asked how she managed to keep herself mentally healthy so that she could care for her girls. Amatruda explained that it is important for the healer to stay healthy herself. She is used to explaining this idea by employing the metaphor of being on an airplane when the oxygen masks come down: "If you are sitting with a child or someone who can't take care of themselves, put on *your* mask first, then take care of them." Selvie-amah appeared baffled by this idea. Amatruda recognized that there was a cultural disconnect here but it is not clear that she saw just how differently she and Selvie-amah understood the impact of trauma. The Western conception of post-traumatic stress held a key assumption that a Sri Lankan might not share: that the mental distress experienced by survivors of horror comes from damage to the individual psyche and that that damage makes it difficult to help others. But, as Fernando's studies showed, Sri Lankans' sense of well-being emanates from their connection to the social network. For a Sri Lankan, the very expression of mental health might be embodied in the act of helping others. To repurpose Amatruda's modern metaphor, putting the oxygen mask over the mouth of the child in the next seat would be the very thing that would allow Selvie-amah to breathe.

Parading Certainties

It is unclear what the Sri Lankans thought of Amatruda, this energetic Western woman lugging her suitcase full of art supplies and Band-Aids into refugee camps. Amatruda reports that she felt welcomed and appreciated. From her perspective the local population certainly seemed to recognize the genuine spirit of caring that brought her to their doorstep in that dark time.

The juxtaposition of these well-meaning Western healers with the devastated landscape was sometimes breathtaking. Here, for instance is how Jennifer Baggerly, an assistant counseling professor at the University of Florida, recounted arriving in the remote village of Kalladi, where 215 families were living in a refugee camp. "The suffering here was clear," she writes. "Rows of white canvas tents in the sweltering sun face a water tank that has been empty for a month and a half. Clean water access is a long walk away so children were thirsty and had unwashed clothes and hair. Some children had a chronic cough while others had sores on their bodies." She then describes her team's psychological intervention, providing "temporary relief from the suffering by conducting our puppet show, helping them make coping bracelets and magazine collages, playing active games, teaching them yoga, and passing out candy and toys to each child."

Dr. Ganesan, who observed many such Western interventions, noted that these relief workers, with their strange behavior, their puppet shows and handcrafts and interactive games, often did liven the mood of the camps they visited. "In many instances these sessions, in which whole communities participated, offered comic relief for the survivors even though it was probably not intended as such," he recalls.

The term "psychosocial aid" has gained great currency among international trauma counselors who like to believe that their interventions are sensitive to cultural differences. In its most promising use, psychosocial aid acknowledges that helping the culture get back to normal functioning is the key to maintaining the mental health of the people. The assumption is that the local people will look to their churches, mosques, schools, and social networks to find support and make meaning of what happened to them. Psychosocial support (again in its most progressive use) suggests that every effort should be made to put these local institutions and networks back in working order so that the people can heal and make meaning in their own way.

In practice, however, it is clear that "psychosocial aid" is often little more than a buzzword. Although many interventions talk of psychosocial aid, local religions and forms of healing are given only lip service or, worse yet, are used as the proverbial spoonful of sugar that helps the Western medicine go down. "Trauma victims in disaster situations may not actively seek mental health services for various reasons," wrote David Surface in *Social Work Today*. "Some may be in denial or simply not aware of the extent to which they've been traumatized, while others may not seek out therapy because of social or cultural stigmas. Therefore, the goal of many disaster mental health workers is to have therapy be seamless, integrated . . . and, whenever possible, incorporate familiar community settings and rituals." In this way of thinking, it is not the community traditions or rituals that are seen as healing but the Western therapy that has been stirred in among local practices.

Some trauma counselors in Sri Lanka all but ignored local custom and practices and stridently asserted that they knew better than the locals how to handle the psychological aftermath of the disaster. William Yule, a child psychologist from King's College in London, expressed with particular certainty that he knew what was best for the population. He reported with concern that orphaned children were sometimes coaxed through the experience by relatives who told them that their parents hadn't in fact drowned but had taken jobs that required them to travel to foreign lands. Yule made it clear that this lack of disclosure would psychologically damage the children. He writes that he had to have long discussions with locals "to clarify . . . the need to be honest with children."

It's true that the period after the tsunami was filled with such hopeful lies and misinformation told not only to orphaned children but often to desperate parents looking for missing offspring. Neighbors or relatives would sometimes tell frantic parents of having seen a missing child or heard that the child had shown up in a neighboring village. Following such rumors, one after the next, some parents traveled hundreds of miles up or down the coast. These well-meaning lies are certainly heartbreaking and clearly go against many assumptions of Western mental health treatment, which values facing and "working through" or "processing" unhappy experiences. But was Yule's insistence that these stories were psychologically damaging a universal truth or a culturally based assumption?

What Yule didn't comprehend was that these sorts of stories are not particular to Sri Lanka or the tsunami. Anthropologists working in poor or war-torn nations have documented similar narratives. Based on her work with Somali refugees, for instance, the anthropologist Christina Zarowsky wrote that if a person goes missing and is almost surely dead, it is socially acceptable to lie to family members to "ease their mind" and say that the missing person has gone abroad. This is a story born of poverty-stricken places where people die young or disappear just as completely through emigration to far-off lands. Dismissing such stories as psychologically beyond the pale ignores the tragic social forces from which they spring. In the end all stories about where parents or children "go" when they die are, to varying degrees, wishful and culturally bound. How, one might reasonably ask, is Yule's insistence on the "need to be honest" in this sad situation any less culturally imperialistic than a Christian missionary trying to disabuse some far-flung population of a local notion of reincarnation?

But regardless of whether trauma counselors tried to be culturally sensitive or, like Yule, paraded their certainties, the result was likely the same. Dr. Siddharth Ashvin Shah, who traveled from his home in the United States to Sri Lanka after the tsunami to try to help, reports that he arrived determined to let local healers take the lead. What he discovered was that the social forces at play made this approach nearly impossible. "The recipients are driven by a belief that they lack things, concepts, and behaviors that the West can supply," Shah recounts. "The non-West craves our technology because it anticipates good innovation from the West. We produce information that verifies its effectiveness. . . . We are confident that we have something exceptional to offer and not the other way around."

Try as he might to be respectful of local beliefs, Shah found that it was impossible to abdicate the role he was expected to fill, that of "Western expert" bringing advanced knowledge. "The attention experts like myself command is triumphalist," he wrote, "blinding the relief workers and myself to the culturally embedded self-concepts and healing practices." As much as trauma counselors talked of "psychosocial approaches" or "cultural competency," the obvious preference given to the Western ideas of psychological suffering often overwhelmed their best intentions.

Global Differences in Suffering

A careful look at other cultures and moments in human history shows that there is little about the human reaction to trauma that is universal. For instance, the assumption that each generation of soldiers reacts the same way to combat is turned on its head by even the briefest look at history. There is no doubt that soldiers often come back from battle with psychological as well as physical injuries; the fear and horror of direct combat can clearly damage the psyche of men and women. But the medical records of war veterans kept over the past centuries show that the manifestation of the injury is always tied up with cultural beliefs contemporaneous to the time. British soldiers in the Boer Wars were likely to complain of joint pain and muscle weakness, a condition their doctors called "debility syndrome." In the American Civil War, soldiers often reacted to the psychological trauma of battle by experiencing an aching in the left side of the chest and having the feeling of a weak heartbeat, labeled "Da Costa's syndrome." Or they experienced a withdrawal and lethargy thought to be a type of pathological nostalgia caused by being far from home. In the First World War, British and American soldiers commonly experienced "shell shock," with symptoms that included nervous tics, grotesque body movements, and even paralysis. So although the potential psychic damage of war is indisputable, the process by which that damage becomes an outward symptom is a reflection of the cultural beliefs in a particular time and place. The unconscious mind of a soldier latches onto culturally current symptoms of distress (chest pain for the Civil War soldier and muscle spasms for the World War I soldier) because those symptoms are recognized as legitimate during a particular time.

It is important to emphasize that even though symptoms change over time, this is not a matter of faking or play-acting on the part of those psychologically traumatized. Rather, soldiers from different times are unconsciously internalizing cultural expectations and then experiencing them as unavoidable and real. The simple but mind-bending truth is that mental illnesses such as PTSD can be both culturally shaped and utterly real to the sufferer. Therefore, as the medical anthropologist Allan Young explained to me, a diagnosis of PTSD "can be real in a particular place and time, and yet not be true for all places and times."

What is true across time is also true across cultures.

Researchers studying psychological reactions to trauma in cultures around the world have found remarkable deviations from the PTSD symptom list. Salvadoran women refugees who endured a protracted civil war, for example, often experience something called *calorias*, a feeling of intense heat in their body. Although these women did experience sleep disturbances, which is one symptom of PTSD, they did not, for the most part, report increased startle responses or other physical reactions when reexposed to symbols of the trauma. For some Cambodian refugees, the most pressing psychological impact of trauma was being visited by vengeful spirits and the accompanying feeling of intense distress that, in escaping from the country, they had not been able to perform rituals for the dead.

"The meaning of a horrible event has a tremendous impact on the human psyche, and that meaning differs across the world," says psychology professor Ken Miller of Pomona College. "The meaning matters as much as the event itself." Applying the same interviewing techniques Fernando used in Sri Lanka, Miller has studied psychological reactions to war trauma in Afghanistan. His analysis yielded many reactions not on the PTSD symptom list, and several that had no ready translation in English. There was, for instance *asabi*, a type of nervous anger, and *fisha-e-bala*, the sensation of internal stress or pressure. The only way for aid providers to be effective, Miller believes, is for them to understand the local idioms of distress—the particular ways psychological trauma is understood, experienced, and expressed in specific cultural contexts.

Duncan Pedersen from McGill University found unique expressions of psychological trauma among the Quechua natives in the southern central Peruvian Andes who were caught up in the brutality of the Maoist guerrilla movement the Shining Path and the Peruvian army. The estimated death toll during the period

topped sixty-nine thousand, with more than half a million internally displaced. The horror they suffered was remarkable both
for its severity and its unrelenting nature. As Pedersen notes, this
was the "destruction of ways of life—targeting and attempting
to eliminate entire ethnic groups, eradicating cultures and social
systems, thus undermining the critical means whereby people can
endure and recover from suffering and loss." The Shining Path
even enforced strict rules for how victims of the conflict were to be
mourned, deeming the traditional public tears of women to be "a
sign of weakness."

Pedersen and his fellow researchers discovered that the people
of the Ayacucho highlands have two distinct semantic categories
to describe their suffering. *Nakary* conveys the notion of collective
suffering, often described with the metaphor "it's like carrying the
cross on the shoulders of everyone," and includes the notion that
this suffering is a punishment for wrongdoings in the past. *Llaki*,
on the other hand, refers to the individual experience of sorrow and
distress. In its extreme form, *llaki* is seen as an illness with symptoms that include a variety of physical pains, such as headaches,
stomach pains, and body aches.

Critically, neither *llaki* nor *nakary* is thought to be related to
specific experiences of trauma or discrete periods of upheaval. These
are experiences of distress indicative of the long-term nature of the
conflict. Because PTSD connects symptoms to specific moments
of trauma, the diagnosis does not take account of the indirect and
ongoing consequences of violence that were most troubling to this
population: the destruction of important social networks and their
webs of reciprocity, the impact on the local economy, the malnutri-
tion, and the spread of disease.

The researchers concluded that the diagnosis of PTSD could
not effectively communicate this type of shared cultural suffering,

"given the multiplicity of ways peoples and societies live through massive trauma, express their distress and suffering, and assign meaning to the human experience." Insisting on employing Western assumptions about trauma, the researchers wrote, potentially "undermined indigenous health systems and largely discredited the power of local healing practices, as well as resiliency, coping and survival strategies." In short, using the PTSD diagnosis and foreign notions of trauma counseling in this situation had the potential to continue, in a new form, the very cultural demolition that had caused the population its greatest distress.

The argument that the insertion of Western PTSD beliefs might actually undercut and disempower the local culture has been made by other researchers as well. In East Timor two researchers, Kathleen Kostelny and Michael Wessells, visited the war-torn area around the capital of Dili and saw a population pushed to the breaking point by war and the increased sexual violence and poverty that came with it. Most distressingly, the Indonesian militias often destroyed or ransacked sacred structures where families and clan members performed rituals and kept their sacred objects. This amounted to a "spiritual calamity," according to Kostelny and Wessells. The insertion of trauma counseling and PTSD didn't ameliorate this problem; it heightened it.

"In a situation of desperation, local people often silence their own cultural practices, cling to Western approaches that have the imprimatur of science, or 'play along' by giving the appearance of accepting outside approaches in hopes of getting food or money from powerful outsiders," Kostelny and Wessells conclude. They note that this undermining of local pathways to recovery can happen so subtly as to escape the notice of both the caregivers and those being provided for. "Tacitly, a damaging message sent is that local views and practices are inferior. In the authors' field experience, this message can strengthen a colonially implanted sense of inferiority and weaken local people's belief that they have the capacity to build their own positive future."

Education or Indoctrination?

Such concerns about the use of PTSD and Western beliefs surrounding trauma have done little to stem the efforts of Western traumatologists to intervene in other cultures after times of crisis. Why, one might reasonably ask, are we so certain that the rest of the world needs our help in this regard?

A look at the one of the first cross-cultural applications of PTSD—in response to the 1995 earthquake in Kobe, Japan—sheds some light on this question. It was only a matter of days after the disaster when a team of PTSD experts from Harvard University arrived in the city to collect data on the psychological damage caused by the quake. As with other international PTSD research that was to come, it was clear from the start that this was far from a dry exercise in epidemiology. The survey and the results were overtly intended to advocate for a dramatic shift in thinking on the part of the Japanese mental health system. The fact that the report was as much a call to arms as an academic document could be seen in its title: "The Invisible Human Crisis."

"The PTSD concept was used to point to the reality of a field of suffering recognized by the more psychologically advanced culture of the United States but ignored in Japan," reported the anthropologist Joshua Breslau, who studied the aftermath of the Kobe quake. Behind this effort to influence the Japanese response to the disaster was a deep certainty commonly shared by traumatologists that the rest of the world doesn't pay nearly enough attention to mental health and that other cultures lack crucial knowledge that Americans possess.

Although undertaken as humanitarian outreach, these efforts often look more like massive attempts at indoctrination. To accept the ideas of PTSD, other cultures first had to be "educated" in the appropriate symptoms of PTSD and modern modes of healing. After the genocidal killings in Rwanda one nongovernmental organization (NGO) quickly produced seventy-five thousand copies of a brochure on the signs and symptoms of traumatic stress. Foreign trauma counselors gave interviews to local journalists on the psychological sequelae of trauma, and public health campaigns were undertaken to educate the benighted population in the symptoms of PTSD. Within two years of the killings more than six thousand "trauma advisors" had been trained in the country. Less than two years later, they reported that more than 144,000 children had been counseled.

Similarly, within hours of the bombing of the U.S. Embassy in Nairobi, Kenya, in 1998, a trauma counseling program called Operation Recovery was put into motion. "Mental health experts used local and national radio and television broadcasts to discuss the symptoms of acute stress reactions, and these broadcasts continued for 2 weeks after the bombing," wrote two psychiatrists of the project. More than seven hundred counselor-trainees were given a two-day seminar on PTSD within a week of the bombings.

An equally impressive intervention came the next year, when trauma counselors went to the mountainous area on the northern coast of Venezuela after a massive flood and landslide claimed more than fifty thousand lives. A radio, TV, and newspaper ad campaign was launched to make the population aware of what psychological consequences to expect, and posters of the PTSD symptom list were placed in schools, community buildings, police stations, churches, and grocery stores.

Often these campaigns seemed to imply that the psychological consequences of trauma were similar to a newly discovered disease, and that local populations were utterly unaware of what happens to the human mind after terrible events. That implicit assumption often left anthropologists shaking their heads in disbelief. It takes a willful blindness to believe that other cultures lack a meaningful framework for understanding the human response to trauma.

"Most of the disasters in the world happen outside of the West," says Arthur Kleinman, a medical anthropologist from Harvard University. "Yet we come in and we pathologize their reactions. We say: 'You don't know how to live with this situation.' We take their cultural narratives away from them and impose ours. It's a terrible example of dehumanizing people."

Once one comprehends the cultural differences in psychological reactions to trauma, the efforts of the Western traumatologists who rush into disaster zones on a few days' notice begin to look somewhat absurd. To drive this point home, Miller asked me to consider the scenario reversed. "Imagine our reaction," he said, "if Mozambicans flew over after 9/11 and began telling survivors that they needed to engage in a certain set of rituals in order to sever their relationships with their deceased family members. How would that sit with us? Would that make sense?"

The Rise of Fearlessness

The mistake in applying Western notions of trauma without consideration for local beliefs goes beyond just being ineffective: there is real danger of doing harm. This lesson should have been learned long before the tsunami in, of all places, Sri Lanka.

For over a year and a half starting in 1996, Alex Argenti-Pillen, now an anthropology professor at University College London, spent time in a poor Sri Lankan village trying to make sense of the local modes of psychological suffering while at the same time documenting the impact of the rising influx of Western ideas about trauma.

In response to the ongoing civil war, organizations such as the UN High Commission for Refugees, UNICEF, Oxfam, and the International Rehabilitation Council for Victims of Torture organized workshops and training seminars in the country, and international trauma specialists spoke about PTSD and Western-style trauma counseling. It was commonly asserted at the time that helping war-torn populations heal from PTSD could slow or stop the cycles of violence. Researching the effects of these efforts in small villages, Argenti-Pillen came to the opposite conclusion. She became concerned that these Western ideas of trauma and healing had the potential to destabilize fragile local truces that existed among families, clans, and ethnic groups.

The social and economic situation in the Sinhalese Buddhist village she studied was indeed dismal. There was desperate poverty, and many local men and boys had been drawn into the civil war between the Sri Lankan government and the separatist Liberation Tigers of Tamil. Many of those drafted into the Sri Lankan army deserted from military service, forcing them to lead itinerant lives to avoid arrest. In addition to the civil war, a violent youth revolt by the Janatha Vimukthi Peramuna between 1988 and 1991 brought on a harsh crackdown by the government. Villagers had been brutalized by literally all sides in these conflicts. Neighbors often informed on each other, leading to kidnapping, torture, and murder.

But as bad as the situation was, Argenti-Pillen was interested in what kept the violence from spinning even further out of control. What were the factors that kept villages from undergoing a conflagration of revenge and ethnic violence such as that seen in Rwanda and Bosnia? In the village she studied, there remained boundaries on the violence. Although many men had been killed, their wives and children were usually left physically unharmed. In the aftermath of the violence, perpetrators were clearly disassociated from their families and revenge killings didn't target relatives. In many cases, the family of the killer and the family of the victim (or the informant and the informed upon) remained living side by side.

Argenti-Pillen documented the villagers' remarkably complex way of talking and thinking about the experience of violence that, in several key respects, contradicted assumptions about PTSD. In the cosmology of these villagers, humans are vulnerable to what they call the "gaze of the wild," the experience of being looked in the eye by a wild spirit, which can take the form of a human being intent on violence. According to this belief it is not witnessing violence that is destructive. Rather, the moments of terror that come from violence leave one vulnerable to being afflicted by the gaze. Struck by such a gaze, one enters an altered state of consciousness and can become violent oneself, behave lasciviously, become physically immobilized, or in other ways step outside of normal modes of social behavior. Somatic symptoms, including chronic headaches, stomach aches, and loss of bodily strength, are also common. Someone in this sort of semitrance may speak in the voice of the spirit or alternate between the perspective of the wild spirit and a human state called *inna barikama*, which roughly translates as "can't stay here." Often those experiencing *inna barikama* will yell for hours variations on "I can't stay," "can't live," "can't be," or they will simply repeatedly moan "Can't."

Those afflicted by the gaze of the wild might also express their distress by "becoming closed off" or having "a terrified heart," which can lead to any number of somatic symptoms, including vomiting and physical aches and pain. These semitrance states are treated in the village with a long and arduous cleansing ritual. Such ceremonies often last up to thirty hours, during which the afflicted person is encouraged to dance, tremble, and speak in tongues at specific times during the ceremony. The rituals themselves are designed to elicit fear. Healers elaborately disguised as wild spirits visit the sick, often in the early hours of the morning, in order to frighten the subject as severely as possible. Often those who complete these cleansings show dramatic recoveries.

Interestingly, it doesn't necessarily require a violent event to spark a terrified heart. Simply speaking directly about a recent act of violence, with words that graphically or emotionally evoke the experience, is also considered potentially pathological. Because most villagers hid in their houses during the periods of intense violence, their experience of terror was largely through what they heard. The shouts of the attackers and the cries of the wounded and tortured were the soundscape of the wild spirits and could bring on the fear-related illness of "a terrified heart." "Just as the soundscapes of violence and civil war affect people, so do the words used to represent this reality," Argenti-Pillen concluded. "In other words, discourses about the wild act as agents of the wild."

Stories or even words describing the violence were considered literally dangerous. Because of this, the community had established a complex set of rules for how villagers are allowed to talk about or remember the violence. Argenti-Pillen had to learn a complex dialect of "cautious words" that allow someone to reference a horrifying event without explicitly bringing it to mind. On examining these local euphemisms, she began to see that they were intentionally replacing words or phrases that might invoke fear or moral anger with those that connote safety and trust. Torture, for example, was evoked with a word that also means a child's mischief.

Unraveling this secret code, Argenti-Pillen filled her notebooks with these euphemisms. "Those and these" meant quarrels and fights. "The confusion and mistakes of people who hurry too much" referred to the brutal civil war. A "place that takes sacrifices" indicated a location where many people died. "Funny nonsense" was a way of invoking the disorientation and confusion of the terrified. To "bother" could mean anything from child abuse to bombing. "Rowdy sons" were the perpetrators of violence.

Argenti-Pillen also noticed that women in the village who had suffered from terrified hearts often took it upon themselves to be the enforcers of such indirect speech. While this use of indirect language could easily be filed under the rubric of "psychological avoidance" in the style of the PTSD diagnosis, that would miss the fact that this local custom had a specific purpose. Only gradually did Argenti-Pillen come to understand that the prohibitions on speech were a kind of "acoustic cleansing" by which people protected themselves and others from spreading the gaze of the wild and avoiding a potentially exponential rise in revenge violence. These people weren't avoiding talking about what had happened to them because they were psychologically blocked or traumatized; rather, they were attempting, as best they could, to keep the violence under control.

There was another local reaction to horrible events that ran counter to the idea of the terrified heart. Some women believed that the atrocities they had witnessed or endured had made them become "fearless." Usually "fearlessness" applied to men who acted violently or *yaka*-like (like an evil spirit), but over the years of the civil war women were increasingly embodying the trait as well. These fearless women attested that they were no longer susceptible to having a terrified heart and that they no longer needed the domestic cleansing rituals. It was these fearless women who often violated the rules of cautious speech. They were said to speak with "sharp tongues" and carelessly. Such women often found themselves socially marginalized by those in the village, seen as akin to wild spirits themselves. Fearless women were likely to intentionally raise their children to be fearless as well. Often sons of such mothers

were the boys who became *yaka*-like, prone to violence and terrifying the community.

Into this delicate and intricate social and psychological landscape began to flow Western ideas about trauma and healing. This
transmission of knowledge was not as direct as it was in the aftermath of the tsunami. No Western counselors set up tents on the
outskirts of Argenti-Pillen's village. Rather, these ideas trickled
down from training programs sponsored by NGOs in Colombo.
Western trauma specialists would train regional health care workers; that knowledge would then flow down to rural health care
workers, who then treated and sometimes trained local villagers in
these methods.

The problem was that the central tenet of Western trauma counseling—that traumatic experiences must be retold and mastered—
ran counter to the local customs regarding the use of euphemistic
speech. Rural health care workers were suddenly insisting that
experiences of trauma be spoken about directly. One Sri Lankan
health care provider told Argenti-Pillen that she had learned from
Western experts that it was important not to allow the traumatized
individual to keep secrets or talk around traumatic events. "There is
a method of talking," she said, "talking with our eyes, our face, with
our whole posture, we must tie them to us. . . . We take the information out of the clients. . . . We put them in a position in which
they can't keep any secrets."

The Western-trained counselors saw it as their job to reorient the
population's beliefs about trauma and healing. Many counselors
expressed certainty that their new counseling methods proved
that the traditional local rituals were ineffective. "A terrified heart
cannot be cured by means of domestic cleansing rituals," one
Western-trained counselor told Argenti-Pillen. "The illness that
has hit the mind can sometimes not be cured even if you danced
a thousand cleansing rituals, let alone one. So, if you don't give

counseling . . . in the correct way, that person will stay in the same condition."

However, it was rarely the women with terrified hearts who were first in line for this new method of counseling. After all, it was their job in the community to ensure that people were circumspect in telling stories of violence. Rather, it was the fearless women, with their penchant for telling unambiguous stories of the violence, who embraced the new healing methods. Whereas from the villagers' perspective fearless women were potentially dangerous, from the perspective of the Western-trained counselors they were "empowered." Not only were fearless women often the first to accept trauma counseling; they were also the first to accept training as counselors themselves.

"While the majority of the community consider fearlessness an aberration . . . the NGO activities now provide an outside legitimization for fearlessness," Argenti-Pillen writes. "The NGOs now support fearlessness as a viable form of sociability."

By encouraging fearlessness and pathologizing the local custom of using ambiguous speech, this intervention was tampering with a delicate social balance. Argenti-Pillen's concern was that Western-style trauma counseling was undermining a fragile social stopgap that kept violence in these tight communities from spiraling out of control. These counselors were playing with fire. "Tales of 'traumatized survivors' fail to provide a much-needed framework in which local techniques for containing violence can be safeguarded," she concludes. "They also fail to assess the potential risks of the introduction of the discourse on trauma to such local techniques." Trauma counseling services had the potential to have the exact opposite effect intended. Instead of ending the social cycles of violence, they were potentially removing the brakes. The risk, she concluded, is that "trauma counseling services will further destabilize a local cycle of containment of major outbreaks of violence."

The American Way to Suffer

It would be hard to overstate the certainty that most Americans currently place in the diagnosis of PTSD. Although it has been officially recognized for only twenty-five years, it is reflexively evoked after school shootings, natural disasters, and terrorist attacks. It has become part of our common parlance and conventional wisdom. With so many soldiers serving in the long-term conflicts in Iraq and Afghanistan, PTSD has become a national touchstone in the debate regarding the costs of war. PTSD is as real in our time as *fisha-e-bala* is to an Afghani, as *calorias* is to a Salvadoran, and as terrified heart is to a Sri Lankan.

It is real, that is, but not timeless.

Looking back at the brief history of the disorder, it is remarkable to see how much it has changed even within a generation. A soldier given the diagnosis today would be hard-pressed to recognize it as the same one that was first formulated in the 1970s for soldiers coming home from Vietnam.

The movement to recognize PTSD began as a political as much as a psychiatric movement. Originally called post-Vietnam syndrome, the idea came out of the hothouse of rap sessions held by Vietnam Veterans Against the War and supervised by antiwar psychoanalysts. Dr. Chaim Shatan, who was codirector of the postdoctoral psychoanalytic training clinic at New York University, was one of the first to help find the professional volunteers to sit in on the rap sessions. In a memo he circulated to colleagues his politics were clear: "This is an opportunity to apply our professional expertise and anti-war sentiments to help some of those Americans who have suffered most from the war."

These psychoanalysts and veterans had no intention of carving out a diagnosis that could be applied to all victims of terrifying events, or even all soldiers who experience battle. The original idea was to show that being a soldier in the Vietnam War was an experience utterly distinct from that of being a soldier in any other military conflict. Listen to one of the first descriptions of post-Vietnam syndrome, written by Shatan and published in the *New York Times* in the spring of 1972. According to Shatan, these veterans felt upset because they had been "deceived, used and betrayed" by both the military and society at large. Although Shatan did mention that these veterans experienced "rage," he did not link this or any psychological reaction to particular traumatic battlefield experiences. Instead the rage, as Shatan described it, "follows naturally from the awareness of being duped and manipulated" by the military and the U.S. government. It was the moral ambiguity of the Vietnam War and the deceitfulness of the U.S. government and military, not the trauma of battle, that damaged the psyche of the soldier.

In their push to gain official diagnostic status in the *DSM*, the advocates for recognition of post-Vietnam syndrome found it necessary to cede some ground. Despite the early arguments intent on carving out a disorder specific to the experience of Vietnam veterans, it proved politically expedient to make alliances with other researchers and clinicians who wanted to extend the concept to include those who suffered psychologically after surviving other horrors, including fires, natural disasters, and accidents. The earlier argument that the psychological trauma suffered by Vietnam veterans was utterly specific to soldiers in that conflict was put aside and then forgotten.

As PTSD expanded in influence, more and more advocates were making the argument that the disorder had an immutable objective existence independent of culture, time, or place. This left the obvious question: If it was so timeless, why had it only recently been recognized?

In a history of the International Society for Traumatic Stress

Studies, written by one of the group's former presidents, Dr. Sandra Bloom, the early advocates of the disorder are portrayed as the first to bravely overcome the social pressure to ignore the psychological reaction to trauma. Forces in our society, Bloom writes, have a stake in "denying the profound and long-term effects of trauma. . . . The larger society will continue to deny the magnitude of the problem not only because of the emotional arousal exposure causes, but because it is becoming increasingly clear that fixing the problems and actually preventing trauma, will cost a great deal." PTSD has always been with us, the argument went, but we were just now raising our consciousness to the point that we could face its devastation.

As the diagnosis expanded in the West, encompassing more and more experiences, there grew a market for those claiming to have the latest techniques for treating the condition. These techniques, in turn, began to shape our cultural expectations and understanding of how trauma affects the mind. Few were more influential in creating the American style of PTSD than a former paramedic named Jeffrey T. Mitchell, who created a seven-step regimen called Critical Incident Debriefing. Mitchell's debriefings were intended to be performed in the first hours or days after a threatening event. Led by a trained facilitator, groups of survivors would be first informed of the common reactions to traumatic stress. Each participant was then encouraged to describe his or her perspective on the trauma in order to "make the whole incident come to life again in the room."

The metaphor of trauma creating a "psychic wound" was taken quite literally. It just made sense that the quicker debriefers got to the scene, the more they could do for the victims. Beginning in the late 1980s counselors armed with this new knowledge were rushed to the scenes of school shootings, train wrecks, fires, maritime disasters, and all manner of other calamity. In 1989 Mitchell founded an organization called the International Critical Incident Stress Foundation to teach debriefing as a method of heading off PTSD. The foundation grew quickly and was soon training tens of thousands of debriefers each year.

The fall of 1989 proved to be a watershed moment for the American public's awareness of trauma counseling and the ideas behind critical incidence debriefing. In September of that year Hurricane Hugo made landfall on the coast of South Carolina, pushing a twenty-foot wall of water over coastal communities. Disaster counseling and critical incident debriefers were included in the response to the devastation, to the fascination of the journalists and public who followed the events.

Just a month later, on the other side of the country, the Loma Prieta earthquake struck the San Francisco Bay Area. Occurring during the pregame warm-up to the third game of the World Series, the quake was broadcast live to the nation. The first pictures of the collapsed section of the Bay Bridge were sent from the Goodyear Blimp, which had been hovering over Candlestick Park to cover the game. Many mental health workers who had been providing debriefing and trauma counseling in the coastal towns of South Carolina got on planes and flew directly to San Francisco to set up counseling services for quake victims. Again, reporters and TV crews focused a great deal of attention on these efforts.

By the time Hurricane Andrew sliced through the southern tip of Florida and crashed into the south central portion of Louisiana three years later, the public's respect for the PTSD diagnosis and the need for trauma counseling had solidified. That new certainty could be heard in a Knight Ridder/Tribune news service story filed in Miami: "Hurricane Andrew's biggest impact wasn't its physical destruction. That was only $20 billion. What it wrought in South Floridians' minds is incalculable." By this point Mitchell's International Critical Incident Stress Foundation was training upwards of thirty thousand debriefers each year.

Despite the public and professional certainty that counselors and debriefers should rush in after disasters to treat traumatized populations, there was one problem: there was little evidence that such efforts helped. In fact study after study published during the 1990s, the heyday of trauma counseling, showed that early interventions were either ineffective or actually caused harm. One study followed several hundred car accident victims over a three-year period. At random, some of the victims were debriefed or given no immediate psychological treatment. Interviewed three years later, victims displayed a remarkable difference: the people who were debriefed were more likely to be anxious and depressed and harbor a nagging fear of riding in cars. The study, which was published in the *British Medical Journal* in 1996, concluded, "Psychological debriefing is ineffective and has adverse long-term effects. It is not an appropriate treatment for trauma victims." Another study of burn victims showed a similar effect: measured after a year, those who had been debriefed were much more likely to qualify for the diagnosis of PTSD and to express hostility, feel depressed and anxious, and report a lower quality of life than those who received no help. The conclusion was that the early interventions were actually impeding the mind's natural healing process.

Early interventions sometimes appeared to be priming victims to experience certain symptoms. "When dealing with people after an accident we need to remember that emotionally aroused people are suggestible," David Brown, a psychologist from Australia, wrote later in the *British Medical Journal*. "If we suggest they might feel angry, it is likely to come true."

Others have noticed the same phenomenon. "Sometimes when we put people in a group and debriefed them, we gave them memories that they didn't have," Malachy Corrigan, the director of the Counseling Service Unit of the New York City Fire Department, told the *New Yorker.* "We didn't push them to psychosis or anything, but, because these guys were so close and they were all at the fire, they eventually convinced themselves that they did see something or did smell something when in fact they didn't."

Looking back, it is remarkable that so little attention was paid to the danger that debriefing might be shaping and suggesting reactions in the minds of distressed individuals. Social psychology has a rich literature on group belief-building and social contagion that could have been well employed here. If you take a group of disoriented and unsettled victims mere hours or days after a life-altering tragedy, put them in a highly charged encounter where they are told to expect certain psychological symptoms, and then they share their experiences, you are creating the perfect setting by which emotions are likely to spread and intensify.

Why didn't these practices cease in the face of the evidence that they might actually be harming those they intended to treat? Dr. Richard Gist of the Kansas City Fire Department, who researched the impact of debriefing, noted that the evidence for and against trauma counseling was beside the point because debriefing was, he told a journalist, "more of a social movement." Indeed the evolution of the ideas behind PTSD and the promotion of modern ideas of trauma counseling have been social movements from the beginning. This fact, however, is seldom acknowledged by the evangelical trauma counselors who travel the world to inform other populations about the modern treatments for PTSD.

It is a psychological truism that those who display dead certainty in their convictions are often hiding or covering up for deep insecurities. Professor Vanessa Pupavac, writing from the School of Politics at the University of Nottingham, links the rise in our international trauma interventions—our confident assertions that we must teach the world how to respond to horrible events—with a period of time when we in the West had become increasingly uncertain about how to help the developing world.

The 1990s was a period when our efforts to help other countries with money and aid began to seem impossibly complex and fraught. Book after book took to task humanitarian efforts for bureaucratic waste, having shortsighted goals, and encouraging dependence. This crisis of confidence in the humanitarian community was, Pupavac argues, a reflection of a deep post–cold war uncertainty at home. We had become, she writes, "bereft of convictions and disposed to introspection. . . . The erosion of previous political or communal affiliations [had] not resulted in a vigorous individualism, but anxious insecure individuals."

When we looked out at the violence and hardship in the rest of the world and knew that our psychological assistance was desperately needed, we may have been simply projecting our own postmodern insecurities.

Trauma Stripped of Meaning

In reading the best anthropological writing on the "idioms of distress" in other cultures, one is often struck by the richness of these psychological and social landscapes. The experience of horror or violence in these places is interwoven into religions, social networks, traditions, and rituals of burial and grieving. When one comes back home to PTSD, the starkness and thinness of the idea become glaringly apparent. In the modern Western world, the idea of PTSD is that of a broken spring in a clockwork brain.

PTSD researchers would certainly object to this characterization. They would point to the tens of thousands of research papers, monographs and books on the topic. How could so much research be characterized as "thin"? But I'm not talking about the research, but rather the experience of the PTSD sufferer. By isolating trauma as a malfunction of the mind that can be connected to discrete symptoms and targeted with new and specialized treatments, we have removed the experience of trauma from other cultural narratives and beliefs that might otherwise give meaning to suffering. Being value-neutral to cultural beliefs is problematic given that these beliefs—be it God's plan for someone who's lost a child or patriotism for the soldier crippled in battle—are the very places where we once found solace and psychological strength.

Think back to the ideas surrounding post-Vietnam syndrome. The original intent of that designation was to create a social narrative to prove that being a soldier in the Vietnam War was different from being a soldier in other wars at other times. Proponents were searching for meaning and coming up with stories of government betrayal and the destruction of social trust. Beliefs that had sustained many of their fathers in World War II were suddenly insufficient and meaningless to these soldiers. They replaced those beliefs with another, angrier set of ideas that might give meaning to their experience. But as it evolved into its modern clinical form, PTSD left behind such quests for social meaning in tragedy. In doing so, it has set adrift those struggling in the aftermath of trauma. In contrast to those angry but socially engaged Vietnam War veterans, the personal accounts of current-day soldiers returning from Afghanistan and Iraq often seem pigeonholed into a PTSD diagnosis that is tied to a particularly modern style of lonely hyperintrospection.

Here's one soldier blogging on a popular website devoted to PTSD:

> I constantly doubt how I feel. I don't know if it's real or if
> I'm making it up. . . . I feel guilty. When I was in the service,

the Air Force therapist said that it was PTSD . . . but I don't know if he was right. I worry that I'm trying to fool everyone, even myself. I didn't do anything. I never fired a weapon in combat. I missed everything, I feel guilty about it, and I feel ashamed that I even consider that PTSD might be the problem. I feel like I don't deserve to think this is what is wrong with me. I can't bring myself to read up on PTSD on the internet, because I'm worried that the more I know about it, the more likely I am to make it be the problem subconsciously. . . . I feel like I've fooled myself into playing a character and I don't know how to just put it down.

PTSD is clearly too narrow a category to give meaning to this soldier's experience, but he worries it like a bone because he doesn't appear to have other options; the frustration, anger, and unhappiness of modern soldiers have been moved from the social (where one might find moral anger, nationalistic justification, or religious meaning to justify the sacrifice) to the biopsychomedical. Because PTSD largely focuses on internal states and chemical imbalances within the individual brain, this explanation for psychological problems often leaves the soldier, to borrow a recent military marketing slogan, feeling like "an army of one."

Looking at ourselves through the eyes of those living in places where human tragedy is still embedded in complex religious and cultural narratives, we get a glimpse of our modern selves as a deeply insecure and fearful people. We are investing our great wealth in researching and treating this disorder because we have rather suddenly lost other belief systems that once gave meaning and context to our suffering.

Patrick Bracken, a senior research fellow at Bradford University's Department of Health Studies, argues that the emergence of PTSD is a symptom of a troubled postmodern world. "In most Western societies there has been a move away from religious and other belief systems which offered individuals stable pathways through life, and meaningful frameworks with which to encounter suffering and death," Bracken writes. "The meaningful connections of the social world are rendered fragile." Although we might be able to ignore the absence of these belief systems during our normal day-to-day lives, truly traumatic events have the power to startle us into awareness of a heart-stopping emptiness. The diagnosis of PTSD can categorize some of our reactions to trauma, but in the end it is cold comfort. It cannot replace what we've lost.

Without social mechanisms to cope, we've become increasingly vulnerable and fearful. Indeed many have pointed out that we are now a culture that has a suspicion of resilience and emotional reserve. "In a momentous shift, contemporary Western culture now emphasizes not resilience but vulnerability," says Derek Summerfield, of Kings College, who has worked extensively with victims of war and genocide. "We've invited people to see a widening range of experiences as liable to make them ill. This becomes a problem because we are globalizing our culture. We are presenting just one version of human nature—one set of ideas about pain and suffering—as being definitive. In truth, there is no one psychology."

The Civil War Reignites

Seven months after the tsunami, Lakshman Kadirgamar, the Sri Lankan foreign minister, was murdered in his home by a sniper. The precarious cease-fire between the government and the separatist rebels began to destabilize. By the end of that year the guerrillas in the north of the country were again fighting the government both on land and at sea. The conflicts escalated until, in January

2008, the government officially withdrew from the cease-fire agreement. The battle in the next year would not go well for the Tamil Tigers. By the end of spring 2009 the government forces had routed the Tamil rebels from their last stronghold.

The reality for the civilian population caught in the fighting on the ground became so grim that Gaithri Fernando found that for the first time she had to avoid all news of her home country. She had heard too many stories of mothers digging shallow graves for their children and families trying to escape the fighting by fleeing deep into the jungle, only to lose family members to animal predators.

In the uneasy peace after the fighting, there was again much interest in psychological healing and the damage of PTSD. Having alerted the Sri Lankan Parliament of the abuses of parachute researchers after the tsunami, Dr. Athula Sumathipala published a series of articles in the *Island* newspaper asking again for restraint on the part of globe-trotting trauma counselors. "Undue emphasis on counseling or medicalizing the psychological, sociological and political implications of the displaced population should not be promoted," he wrote. "What [the displaced populations] need is not 'therapy' but provision of basic needs, care with dignity, respect, reassurance to avoid uncertainty and move them to accommodation as soon as possible so that they will have some privacy and also the opportunity to reintegrate to 'normal' life. The best therapy will be a sound social policy."

Whether his voice will be heard is not yet clear. Thanks to the many training seminars set up after the tsunami, there are now thousands of Sri Lankans who believe they are trained in trauma counseling and the Western ideas behind PTSD. In addition, there will undoubtedly be new efforts by international aid agencies to provide psychological therapy. Whether these efforts will heal these communities or, as Argenti-Pillen fears, unintentionally destabilize them remains to be seen. It would be tragic and ironic if Western-style trauma counseling ends up sparking violence between ethnic groups and clans that already have reason to hate each other. Intending to break cycles of violence, Western beliefs about trauma and healing may be poised to spin them back into motion.

The Shifting Mask of Schizophrenia in Zanzibar

What we say about mental illness reveals what we value and what we fear.

JULI MCGRUDER

On my first night in Zanzibar I was awakened by the distant sound of a telephone ringing. I came to consciousness fitfully, puzzling out where I was. I was bone-tired from two days of red-eye plane travel and a rough ferry crossing to the island from mainland Tanzania, disoriented by the ten-hour time change and, possibly, by the side effects of the prophylactic malaria medication I had begun taking a few days before. I checked the bedside clock: 3 a.m. I could hear my hosts, Juli McGruder and her partner, Ahmed Kassim, in the upstairs room of the house as one of them answered the phone. As in most houses in Zanzibar, there was no glass in the windows—better to let the steady trade winds sweep out the stuffy air during the night—and I could hear their voices talking low and intently in Kiswahili. I stood at the window, listening and looking out into the night. It was a full moon and there was a racket of premorning birdsong coming from the thick, low brush beyond the cinderblock wall that surrounded the house. After a few minutes Kassim came downstairs, walked across the sandy driveway, and drove off in his rattletrap Toyota van. I got back in bed, retucked the mosquito netting, and lay awake wondering what might have occasioned the call. I was new to the local customs, but I suspected that Americans and Zanzibaris shared at least this cultural truism: no good news comes in a phone call at 3 a.m.

I had come to Zanzibar, a sixty-mile long coral island off the Swahili coast of East Africa, to spend some time with McGruder. She had recently retired from her teaching position at the University of Puget Sound in Washington and had opened a guesthouse at the very northern tip of the island with Kassim, a younger local man who was both her romantic and her business partner. She had been a professor of occupational therapy, and late in her career she had received a PhD in anthropology from the University of Washington. Her field research focused on three families struggling with schizophrenia in Zanzibar, where she went to figure out a puzzle that has baffled cross-cultural researchers in mental illness for twenty years: Why did people diagnosed with schizophrenia in developing nations have a better prognosis over time than those living in the most industrialized countries in the world?

In the morning I met McGruder in the kitchen, where she was brewing a pot of strong cowboy coffee, boiling the grounds directly in a pot of water. "I need the real thing this morning," she said by way of greeting. "Instant is not going to do it." She told me the news before I could ask. The early morning phone call had been for Kassim. His 10-year-old daughter, Latifa, a child from an early marriage, had died suddenly in the night. The family had known that the girl had an enlarged heart, but she had recently been healthy and happy. Just that day she had been to Koran school, played with her friends, and eaten well. But that night she woke up vomiting blood. The family had rushed her to the hospital, where she died shortly after being admitted. Kassim had gone south to assist with the burial, which, according to Muslim custom, would happen that day.

After a moment I asked how Kassim was holding up. McGruder shrugged as she stirred the coffee. "It's hard to say," she said. "Swahili men tend not to show a lot of emotion when things like this happen."

When I saw Kassim late the next day, I shook his hand and told him how sorry I was to hear about his daughter. He smiled weakly and said only, "That is life." Later at dinner he told McGruder and me how the women cried during the day. He described how the crying would reach a crescendo and then die down, only to be started again when a new woman showed up and saw the body.

Kassim's own demeanor remained a mystery to me. At first I assumed that he was just in shock and would be overcome with emotion when he had time to reflect on the event. It would be unfortunate, I also found myself thinking, if some notion of local machismo made him push his true feelings aside. He would certainly pay a steep psychological price for such repressing of his feelings.

Although I had traveled here with the intention of learning about the different ways people in Swahili culture express emotion in the face of mental illness and other difficult life challenges, I couldn't let go of my assumption that the healthy reaction to the loss of a child would be abject displays of grief. I believed the natural—the truly human—reaction to such an event was the way I imagined I would have reacted if the 3 a.m. phone call had carried tragic news about my own daughter back in San Francisco. I was as unable to understand what Kassim was feeling from his outward affect as I was to understand the meaning of his words when he spoke Kiswahili; he was expressing himself in an emotional language that I did not comprehend.

Even anthropologists, who diligently train themselves to be nonjudgmental observers of cultural differences, have trouble when it comes to recognizing and allowing for cultural differences in emotions. Because our emotions come into our consciousness unbidden and often surprise us with their intensity, we often assume that they are not influenced by cultural cues or social scripts. But with careful study, anthropologists have learned that emotions are not like muscle reflexes; rather, they are communications with deep and sometimes obscure meanings. Cultures differ not only in their response to specific events (as we've seen with reactions to trauma) but also in more global ways.

Describing and understanding these differences has in fact been central to McGruder's research on Zanzibari families who struggle with schizophrenia. During her research she began to suspect that the emotional tenor of families dealing with mental illness in Zanzibar was qualitatively different from that of families in the industrialized world. Subtle differences in this emotional temperature of households, she theorized, might go a long way to explaining why a schizophrenic patient in Zanzibar will often do better than someone diagnosed with the disease in the United States.

From the Clouds to the Equatorial Sun

McGruder is of a type common among the faculty of West Coast colleges. Her politics are liberal and she is prone to antiestablishment and contrarian thinking. She is short with spiked blond hair and a friendly but no-nonsense demeanor. As a child she was smart and rebellious, a difficult combination for a Catholic schoolgirl growing up in northern Indiana in the 1950s. When she was a teenager she dated African American men despite her parents' strenuous objections. One of her first encounters with the mental health profession was when her parents forced her to see a psychologist to cure her of her "pathological" romantic behavior. At one point she was even threatened with incarceration in a mental hospital.

Despite her parents' efforts, she got married at age 18 to an African American man. This was just one year after the Supreme Court's 1967 ruling *Loving v. Virginia*, which effectively ended race-based restrictions on marriage in the United States. McGruder's first job after college was in the mid-1970s at the Hudson River Psychiatric Center in Poughkeepsie, where she witnessed what passed for mental health treatment at the time. As she remembers, the doctors relied heavily on sedating antipsychotics such as Thorazine, Stelazine, and Haldol and some early tricyclic antidepressants. She couldn't help but notice the way some of the drugs knocked the patients for a loop. "These drugs worked like big hammers," she told me. "They just snowed people. They would make the patients shake and drool and feel miserable."

After that she went back to school for a degree in science education and became a teacher, eventually finding a post teaching occupational therapy at the University of Puget Sound. On the side she worked as a private therapist and guardian with elderly and institutionalized schizophrenic clients. After a decade of teaching and making her way up the university's academic ladder, she got bored with the routine and found herself reading feminist philosophical tracts on science and gender. With a sabbatical coming up, she sent out dozens of letters to international aid agencies offering her services. For months she heard nothing. Then came a lone reply from a Danish international development organization that had an office in Dar es Salaam, Tanzania. They offered her a year-long post at the Kidongo Chekundu Mental Hospital on the island of Zanzibar with a salary of forty-two dollars a month. She jumped at the chance and immersed herself in learning Kiswahili. Once she got to Zanzibar, she helped establish an occupational center at the hospital where patients could learn carpentry skills and practice art therapy.

The Western-trained doctors she met at the hospital in Zanzibar had access to the basic arsenal of Western antipsychotic drugs. However, the idea that diseases such as schizophrenia spring from chemical imbalances or brain abnormalities had not yet been accepted by most of the population of Zanzibar. Much more salient were beliefs in spirit possession and the permeability of the human consciousness by magical forces.

McGruder became fascinated by the ways these beliefs in spirits shaped the experience of mental illness both for the families and the patients themselves. She was also interested in how these local ideas were beginning to intermingle and sometimes compete with the imported Western idea that mental illnesses were caused by biological brain malfunctions. At the end of her sabbatical, she decided to pursue a doctoral degree in anthropology so she could dive further into these questions. After finishing her course work in anthropology at the University of Washington, she couldn't wait to escape the dreary Pacific Northwest and get back to the island.

Zanzibar lies at the midpoint of the Swahili Coast, a 1,800-mile stretch of coastline straddling the Equator from Kenya to Mozambique. For millennia it was to this coastline that all of Central Africa brought its goods in order to trade them with the world. The predictable monsoon trade winds were key to its culture. From November to March those winds blew steadily down the coast, bringing merchants and traders from India and the Persian Gulf. From July to September they shifted northward, sending the traders home. On the northbound winds small lateen-sailed boats called dhows traveled up the coast with sturdy mangrove wood, aromatic tree resins, gold, ivory, clove, and the fine, multipurpose fibers of the raffia palm. On the southbound winds they brought back manufactured goods from Arabia, India, and China in the form of carpets, incense, glassware, and cloth. The months between the shifts in the trade winds gave merchants from the Middle East time to sell their goods and buy their new cargo. It also gave them time to share their ideas and religious beliefs and to infuse Swahili with Arabic words. The months in foreign harbors also allowed for merchants and sailors to take wives and otherwise leave their genetic mark on the population.

The resulting cultural texture of Zanzibar was endlessly interesting to McGruder. She enjoyed the smell and the sound of the place, the way the echoing calls to prayer broke up the day, and the constant commotion of children at play. She even liked the way the names of things felt on her tongue. The place-names Kisimkazi, Manzi Moja, and Kakunduchi felt good to say. She particularly liked saying the name of the local public transport along one of the main roads: the *Bububu daladala*.

Not that life there was a tropical paradise. Although her memory of that first year has sweetened, her field notes attest to the frustrations of living in a developing country. There were outbreaks of cholera, and the dust whipped up by the constant trade winds during the dry season often contained enough bacteria to cause epidemics of conjunctivitis. Raw sewage sometimes fouled the white beaches and the baby-blueness of the ocean. Fishermen had recently taken to using sticks of dynamite to fish the reefs, and the joy of speaking the words *Bububu daladala* was offset by the sheer terror she felt while actually riding these speeding minibuses.

In the end, however, her desire to return and study mental illness in Zanzibar came not simply out of an abstract pursuit of knowledge or the social good that might come of her findings, but because she felt a deep affinity for the people and the place.

Incidental Content versus Essential Form

McGruder was well aware that the cutting-edge research on schizophrenia was not coming out of the field of anthropology. More than any other mental illness in the Western world, this one belonged to the "hard scientists" who looked for the causes in bad genes, biochemistry, and the structure of the brain. The advent of brain scans—allowing a researcher to see into the head of live patients—brought with it a seemingly endless series of theories about the root cause of the illness. Abnormalities supposedly key to schizophrenia have been reported in the frontal cortex, the prefrontal cortex, the basal ganglia, the hippocampus, the thalamus, the cerebellum—and pretty much every other corner of the brain as well. No firm consensus had emerged about the location or cause, but there was wide agreement that the exciting advances in understanding the disease were coming from the laboratories of brain researchers.

Although far from the limelight, there were scholars and researchers looking at the disease from other perspectives as well. McGruder found perplexing data and fascinating theories in cross-cultural studies of the disease. Although something approximating schizophrenia could be found in populations at every corner of the globe, there were enough variations to suggest that the disease was shaped by something besides the purely genetic or biological.

The most obvious differences between cultures were in the delusions and hallucinations experienced by those with schizophrenia. These harrowing visions and disembodied voices were often distorted reflections of the phobias and fascinations of specific cultures. No one, after all, endures the psychotic delusion that the CIA is beaming microwave signals into his or her fillings unless that person is culturally acquainted with the CIA, modern dentistry, and the disquieting idea that our bodies are constantly permeated by unseen electromagnetic waves.

Those who have studied these differences have noted, among other things, that delusional guilt is most often associated with Judeo-Christian cultures, as are religious hallucinations such as hearing the voice of God. Such hallucinations are rarer in Islamic, Hindu, and Buddhist populations. Schizophrenic patients from Pakistan are more likely to have visual hallucinations of ghosts and spirits than are British schizophrenics, who are more prone to hearing persecuting voices. In traditional Southeast Asian villages, where it is often frowned upon to strive willfully for personal status, delusions of grandeur are rare. In the United States, where celebrity, wealth, and power are popular fetishes, people with schizophrenia commonly believe that they are famous or all-powerful.

It is also clear that delusional content in any particular culture can change over time. In Austria, to take one example, cases of delusions of grandeur, hearing the voice of God, and feeling persecuted have been steadily increasing over the past fifty years, while delusional guilt and psychotic hypochondria are on the decline.

Researchers who focused on the biomedical or genetic linchpins of the disorder often dismissed these differences. The fact that the "delusions of schizophrenics in industrialized societies will concern television sets and x-rays rather than ghosts and spirits . . . [is] often considered to be of secondary importance," writes Rutgers professor of psychology Louis Sass. "They are presumed to have little to do with the illness's genesis or essential form."

Does it really matter that a person with schizophrenia in one culture talks with a dead relative, while someone in another culture believes he is receiving communications from an extraterrestrial? The distinction that often gets made in this debate is between *pathoplastic* aspects of the disease, which vary from person to person, and the *pathogenic* cause, which is assumed to be the root cause of the disorder. Pathoplastic symptoms are often dismissed for describing only the coloring and content of an illness but not its fundamental nature. The true prize—the quest of the brain researchers—was to get past the cultural noise and discover the pathogenic factors that are the universal cause of the illness. They wanted to weed out the "incidental content" and get to the "essential form."

But McGruder kept coming across research suggesting that culture and social setting play a more complicated role in the disease than simply influencing the content of the delusions. Studies showed, for instance, that prevalence rates vary from place to place. Those living in urban settings in the United States and Europe appear to suffer more often from the disease than those living in the country or the suburbs. These curious spikes in the disorder remain even when researchers took migration, drug use, and poverty out of the equation. Men living in the most densely populated areas of Sweden, for instance, are at a 68 percent higher risk of being admitted for psychosis—often the first sign of schizophrenia—than those who live in the countryside. For women the risk is 77 percent higher. Something about city living seems to spark the harrowing delusions, hallucinations, and disorganized thinking characteristic of a schizophrenic break. Stranger still, some neighborhoods in cities produce more schizophrenics, to such a degree that scientists have wondered about the environmental pathogens that might exist in one place and not another.

The more McGruder read of the cross-cultural research on the disorder, the more it appeared to shape-shift from place to place, and no one seemed to have a clear explanation for this. Janis Hunter Jenkins and Robert John Barrett, two of the premier researchers in the field, describe the general state of affairs.

In sum, what we know about culture and schizophrenia is . . . [that] culture is critical in nearly every aspect of schizophrenic illness experience: the identification, definition and meaning of the illness during the primordial, acute, and residual phases; the timing and type of onset; symptom formation in terms of content, form, and constellation; clinical diagnosis; gender and ethnic differences; the personal experience of schizophrenic illness; social response, support, and stigma; and perhaps most important, the course and outcome with respect to symptomatology, work, and social functioning.

By "course and outcome," Jenkins and Barrett are referring to that most perplexing finding in the epidemiology on the disease: people with schizophrenia in developing countries appear to do better over time than those living in industrialized nations.

McGruder read with fascination the startling results of two huge international studies carried out by the World Health Organization over the course of twenty-five years starting in the late 1960s. These two studies, which had follow-up periods of two and five years, took place in a dozen sites around the world, taking into account ten countries and following more than a thousand patients from both rural and urban settings. What they found was that those diagnosed with schizophrenia living in India, Nigeria, and Columbia often experienced a less severe form of the disease (had longer periods of remission and higher levels of social functioning) than those living in the United States, Denmark, or Taiwan. Whereas over 40 percent of schizophrenics in industrialized nations were judged over time to be "severely impaired," only 24 percent of patients in the poorer countries ended up similarly disabled.

That result, which is perhaps the most famous finding in the field of cross-cultural psychiatry, was widely discussed and debated in part because of its obvious irony: the regions of the world with the most resources to devote to the illness—the best technology, the cutting-edge medicines, and the best financed academic and private research institutions—had the most troubled and socially marginalized patients.

McGruder found it remarkable that even in the face of these cross-cultural differences in outcome, some researchers still seemed uninterested. As with the differences in the content of the delusion, these variations in course and outcome were considered in some quarters to be beside the point. Ignoring the WHO studies might make sense to a brain scientist or geneticist looking for the first trigger for schizophrenia, but for someone like McGruder, who had worked closely with and cared for schizophrenic patients, there was nothing—save a miracle cure—more important than the question of the disease's course and outcome.

As McGruder read more about the WHO studies she became fascinated by the debate within psychiatry over the possible reasons for these differences. Some researchers suggested that the demands placed on a person in a poorer nation to be productively employed were lighter and easier to meet. Perhaps there were more opportunities to feel productive by engaging in work with one's family, such as gardening and child care. Others put forward the idea that the expectations for appropriate behavior were clearer and simpler in nonindustrialized, traditional, or premodern cultures. The rules of behavior for living in the modern world simply overwhelmed schizophrenics, causing them increasing distress. Perhaps, suggested others, it was traditional beliefs in supernatural agents and spirit possession that removed the weight of blame and guilt from both the person experiencing psychosis and the family. Still another set of scholars thought that families in certain cultures might express less highly charged attention and criticism toward the ill family member. This research into what was called "expressed emotion" suggested that schizophrenics often got worse when surrounded by family members who were constantly critical of their behavior or showed intense and intrusive concern about their condition.

Given all the different theories that attempted to explain the WHO studies, McGruder could immediately see one truth: no one had yet found a convincing explanation for the cross-cultural differences. Indeed the researchers who conducted the WHO studies admitted as much. Although a "strong case can be made for a real pervasive influence of a powerful factor which can be referred to as 'culture,'" one of the WHO researchers concluded, none of the WHO studies was designed to "penetrate in sufficient depth" to understand what might be happening. This left researchers guessing which cultural factors might be ameliorating this devastating disease.

The fact that researchers couldn't offer meaningful or specific conclusions about the effect of different cultures on schizophrenia didn't surprise McGruder. Culture, as she was learning to understand it as an anthropologist, did not exist in large data sets. The word can be defined in broad terms as, say, the "the intellectual, moral, and aesthetic standards prevalent in a community" or as the "shared symbols and meanings that people create in the process of social interaction." Yet anthropologists firmly hold that culture can be truly understood only in the particular. Culture, especially as it shapes and informs the consciousness of a mentally ill person, is a local phenomenon.

Again and again in the debate surrounding the WHO study McGruder saw researchers pleading for anthropologists to pick up the ball and run. "More ethnography is needed," concluded one well-known researcher, "if only to elucidate those aspects of everyday practice that remain obscure." All the way back in 1987 the Harvard medical anthropologist Arthur Kleinman wrote with obvious frustration about the lack of anthropological attention to the WHO data on schizophrenia: "For over ten years this finding has been the most provocative to emerge in cross-cultural psychiatry . . . [Yet] the most important finding of cultural difference—arguably the single most important finding in the study—receives scant attention."

McGruder saw the window of opportunity presented by the WHO study. What was clearly missing was an on-the-ground examination of the ways patients in a developing country are treated by their families and caregivers. What ideas and beliefs do family members in developing nations use to understand the delusional behavior of a loved one? How do they talk about this behavior—what specific words and ideas do they employ? And, critically, how does the local understanding of the illness impact the beliefs, behaviors, and self-conception of the ill family member?

Given the importance of the questions posed by the WHO studies, it was surprising that droves of young anthropologists hadn't heeded the call. Then again, considering the scope of the challenge, this reticence is perhaps understandable. Even observable public aspects of culture are difficult to understand and describe in depth; elucidating the cultural currents that affect the functioning of a mentally ill person would be much more difficult. The challenge of McGruder's research went beyond describing what people did. She had to explain, on a nearly existential level, who they were. A younger PhD candidate would have been well advised to pick a topic that had firmer boundaries. Fortunately McGruder was not at the beginning of her career but closer to its end, and so she had no need for a safe research topic. She brought to her research the particular type of passion that comes when one picks a topic that is the confluence of one's life interests.

Revolution and Madness

On my fourth day in Zanzibar, McGruder walked me through a maze of narrow alleys in Stone Town to the house of one of the three families she studied. It was a low white building facing a small public square, in the center of which stood a large shade tree. The house was not much to look at: a single-story cement structure with four square columns supporting the roof over a small porch. The windows were shuttered behind steel bars. The family had moved a few years ago and the house was empty. A message in red spray paint read in Kiswahili, "This house is not for sale." This, McGruder told me, was where Hemed and his daughter Kimwana, both diagnosed with schizophrenia, had lived with their family.* The head of the household was Amina, Hemed's ex-wife and Kimwana's mother.

As with most Zanzibari families, these three did not live as a nuclear family unit. During the year McGruder spent visiting the family, the household included Amina's mother; her two married daughters and their children; one unmarried daughter, who was sometimes away at college; one unmarried son, who was studying at the local Islamic teacher's college; Hemed's half-brother, who was a deaf-mute; plus his adopted sister and her children. At night the 600-square-foot, eight-room structure slept as many as ten adults and ten children.

As we sat on a low brick wall at the edge of the square nearest the house, I asked McGruder if her memory of the place was of rooms constantly packed with people. "No, my impression of the place was of traffic; constant streams coming and going," she told me. She described how women would converse and do chores indoors or in

---

*All the names of the African families mentioned in this chapter are pseudonymous.

the small walled courtyard. Men and children would be outside on the covered *baraza*, the cement bench that ran along the front of the house. The kitchen would be in constant use, as household members cared for and fed each other in a bustle of steady activity. One of McGruder's favorite words in Kiswahili is onomatopoeic for such managed chaos: *zogozogo*.

The sheer number of people in the household posed a challenge to her research. She had hoped to tell the history and take the emotional temperature of the family, but even a rough sketch of the family tree of this pulsing kinship group proved complicated. Amina, the mother, seemed the obvious focal point for her study. The swirl of activity in the household revolved around her. She was the rock.

Like many Zanzibaris, Amina was of mixed Swahili and Arab descent. She was married at 18 in an arranged union to Hemed, the older son of the plantation owner for whom her father worked. Like many Arab families who had immigrated from the Middle East over the centuries, Hemed's father owned a clove plantation and traded in the spice business. During their courtship in 1960 and the months after their marriage that year, Amina remembered, Hemed was lighthearted and charming. Sadly, it was less than a year after their marriage that he experienced his first psychotic episode.

The period in which Hemed began to experience symptoms of schizophrenia was, not coincidentally, a time of political upheaval on the island. After years of being a British colony, Zanzibar embarked on the uncertain path to self-governance. There were three political parties, twenty-two trade unions, and sixteen partisan newspapers stirring up anger and resentment on all sides. Hemed's first experience of derangement, McGruder believes, was sparked by the social upheaval of the time.

As Amina remembered, Hemed loved to talk politics, and he would often come back from political meetings so wound up that he couldn't sleep. He would talk all night about the various faction leaders and the ever-changing alliances. Over the months, these ramblings became tinged with fear of political persecution. His worries were not mere paranoia, given the ethnic and political killings that were to come.

Soon Hemed's political monologues transformed into fretful discussions with unseen interlocutors. He began to frighten his new wife with his unpredictable behavior.

Such an onset of schizophrenia can be explained by the stress-diathesis model, the theory that biological factors make one vulnerable to schizophrenia, but stress in one's environment may set off the illness. Stress may come from any number of sources, but researchers have paid particular attention to conflict within a person's social world. Given what was going on in that moment in the history of Zanzibar, the amount of stress felt by Hemed must have been intense. He was a middle-class man from a high-profile Arab minority at a time of growing racial and class distrust. His curly dark hair and facial features made him identifiably Arab. There seemed to be no safe political refuge. Even the political party he belonged to, the Zanzibar Nationalist Party, was internally split between those who considered themselves African and those of Arab heritage. No one knew whom to trust.

At the end of the year Hemed broke down. Soon after his first son was born, in September, he was admitted to the local mental hospital after beating his great-aunt during a delusional episode. Early the next year he was certified as a person of unsound mind. His medical charts reported that he had a "shallowness of emotion, visual hallucinations and aggressiveness, tend[ed] to lose temper, ha[d] delusions."

The New Year brought no relief from the political turmoil. Violent riots followed the elections, prompting the British to send in soldiers from the mainland and declare a state of emergency. Dozens of foreign-born Arabs were murdered and more than a thousand people were arrested. During this time Hemed returned to the mental hospital and stayed there for six months. He was released around the time his daughter Kimwana was born.

Over the next two decades Hemed was hospitalized eight times for various periods and twice given electroconvulsive treatments. As McGruder examined his hospital records, it became clear that the dates of his worst episodes were during or right after periods of political strife or family stress.

In 1970, when Hemed was hospitalized for nearly an entire year, Amina divorced him, employing an Islamic law that allows divorce for reasons of nonsupport. Still, Hemed eventually came back to live with the family, and he and Amina even had a sixth child together. Later he suffered a stroke that paralyzed one side of his body. In the end Amina saw Hemed's stroke as something of a blessing. Although it made him an invalid, she told McGruder, "it has broken the strength of his anger, his wanting to beat people."

Kimwana, their daughter, showed no signs of the illness during childhood. Amina remembers her daughter's early years with the compliment that she was "not a heavy load." She was a happy child even though her early years were turbulent times for the island. Her mother and classmates remember her as the brightest student in the class. Particularly skilled with numbers, she graduated from secondary school and took a job with the Ministry of Finance. This was 1983, a time of rapid change for women on the island. To fill in for the many educated men who had fled the political upheaval, women were beginning to enter the professional workforce by the thousands.

One Saturday night, just a few months after starting her new job, Kimwana was restless and couldn't sleep. Late in the evening she wandered outside the house and in a loud voice began asking for forgiveness. "Forgive me!" she yelled. "Oh God, what have I done wrong!" When the family couldn't calm her, they assumed it was a case of spirit possession. The family debated two theories. Perhaps, they thought, she had been possessed by a spirit from a deceased ancestor who had not been acknowledged for watching over Kimwana, had not been shown the proper gratitude for all the success she had experienced up to that point. The other possibility was that a jealous coworker had sent the spirit with the use of witchcraft.

At 1 a.m. Kimwana's ranting hadn't yet subsided, and the family took her to the local hospital. Amina remembers that she was examined, given antimalaria pills, and admitted for four days.* At the end of the week, Amina recalls, Kimwana came back home, slept well, and was able to go to work again on Sunday.

She worked that week, but the following Monday again became upset and refused to go to work. This time Amina employed a traditional remedy. She burned a mixture of leaves, flowers, grasses, and seaweed, whose strong odor is believed to repel many types of weak spirits. Amina remembers taking her daughter to the hospital, where she again "became herself." But even with periods of remission, the delusions of hearing disembodied voices came back on a regular basis.

He Sees Me up to My Heart

Fifteen years later, when McGruder began to spend time with the family, her goal was not to show that Kimwana's or Hemed's men-

---

*When McGruder compared Amina's memory to the records in the hospital, there were considerable differences. The pills she had been given were not, according to the chart, antimalaria medication but an antispasm drug called trihexyphenidyl hydrochloride, used to counter facial muscle spasms that can be a side effect of a powerful antipsychotic called fluphenazine that had been given to Kimwana in an injection.

tal illness would have had a different course in a different cultural setting; that would be impossible to prove as there are no control groups in ethnographic scholarship. Rather, she set about trying to record how cultural beliefs and practices contributed to the family's understanding of the illness and to their treatment of Kimwana and Hemed.

McGruder first wanted to get an idea of what the experience of madness felt like. Hemed was so disabled by his schizophrenia and the stroke that it was not possible to get a sense of what was happening in his mind. Kimwana, however, had periods of relatively high functioning and could tell McGruder her impressions.

Kimwana told McGruder that the voices she heard in her head were usually male, and they spoke to her as if they could "see to my very soul." These voices told her variations on the theme of what a bad person she was. Sometimes she heard two or more men gossiping that she was a disloyal and disrespectful daughter and sister. The chorus could be relentless: "She doesn't love her mother," one voice would say to the other. "She doesn't love her brothers and sisters. She is not a person of God, just a useless person." Sometimes they would curse her in riddles or make negative but oblique statements such as "Abhorrent badness even to the soul."

Although Kimwana understood that her thoughts were unstable and disorganized, she often insisted the voices were of real people and not delusional. And although she sometimes believed that the voices came from outside the window, her subjective experience was that the person speaking was seeing into her thoughts and feelings. "I don't see him but he does [see me]," she told McGruder. "He really sees me a lot. Actually he sees me up to my heart, up to my mind. He has the ability to speak to me because he is able to see me because whatever I think about he sees it."

Much of the torment of having these male presences in her head related to Islamic rules of female modesty. While the voices were with her, she felt she must respect the codes of conduct as if she were actually in the presence of a man. At such times she could not bathe or undress and she tried not to go to the bathroom. Although she sometimes found it helpful to argue with the voices when they became critical, her sense of decorum made it difficult for her to do this out loud.

This sense of decorum also made Kimwana reluctant at first to name her tormentors, for it turned out that she recognized the voices. They were, she admitted to McGruder, the voices of the bicycle repairmen who worked in front of the house. This bit of reality left McGruder in a quandary over Kimwana's perceptions. For most of the day and often into the evening the voices of the bicycle repairmen could be heard quite clearly in the house. It was often difficult to tell to what extent Kimwana's delusions were jumping off of actual conversations drifting through the window and to what extent they existed exclusively in her mind.

That Kimwana's delusions would come in the form of intrusive auditory hallucinations made sense given the location of the household. The roiling, pulsing sound that filled the square during the day was remarkable for its volume, texture, and complexity. Across the square from the house was the Bakathrir Muslim School for Girls, and directly to the right of the house was the Al Nour Islamic School for Boys. At any given moment the undulating, overlapping choruses of hundreds of children chanting in Arabic could be heard.* The noise that emanated from the schools created a kind of hypnotic background sound, like breaking surf.

On top of that sound could be heard the single voices of individual children teasing and playing with each other or calling out to people in the courtyard. Then there were the voices and footsteps of

---

*I've placed an audio recording of the sound of the square on www.crazy likeus.com if you'd like to listen to the soundscape Kimwana lived in.

adults heading across the square on their errands and the constant squawk of crows in the shade tree. In that cacophony of sounds reverberating and echoing off tin roofs and cement surfaces, the only discernable individual voices were those of the bicycle repairmen chatting among themselves or with their customers as they did their work.

Considering the additional commotion of the comings and goings of the members of the household, the noise must have been unrelenting. The many small children, though well behaved in the manner of most Zanzibari children, created a racket. Hemed, even though he could not walk or even bathe himself, could yell and often did for long stretches without ceasing. Several of the family members shared with McGruder their belief that the noise itself was exacerbating Kimwana's illness. Bimkubwa, the most Westernized of the siblings, told McGruder that Europeans have much smaller families and that their houses were much quieter. "There are too many of us and this place is too noisy," she said emphatically.

Kimwana often asserted that she felt better when she was alone. But given her auditory hallucinations and the general noisiness of her surroundings it was clear that she was talking not just about a desire for physical solitude but also for quiet. "I do like being on my own," she once told McGruder. "Being with people I feel like I am tangled with them. I feel like calming myself, just silently. Just quiet and silent." Unfortunately time alone was a scarce commodity in the packed household. And silence was all but unavailable.

The Emotional Temperature of the Household

It didn't take long for McGruder to sense that Amina's family displayed an amazing tolerance for the difficulties of having two severely mentally ill people (not to mention a deaf-mute) in their household. It was a testament to the strength of this family unit that Hemed, even after the divorce for nonsupport and the years of violent psychotic episodes, was still taken care of by Amina and the family.

McGruder noted that the family took a remarkably relaxed stance toward Kimwana's illness in particular. When asked about Kimwana's symptoms, Amina gave matter-of-fact answers. When McGruder wanted to know what Amina thought of Kimwana's central delusion, all she could elicit was the simple declaration that her daughter felt that the "bicycle repairmen concern themselves with her affairs." Amina told McGruder that she did not share her daughter's belief, but there was no judgment or frustration attached to the delusions. To many questions Amina would only answer, "I am unable to know" or "I take it as one of God's mercies, one of God's wishes."

To try to give me a sense of the emotional tone in this house, McGruder recounted a day in late September after a particularly difficult few months for the household. Kimwana was recovering after taking an overdose of her medication, and a bad cold had sickened nearly everyone in the family. Amina had admitted to McGruder that they were too poor even to buy aspirin. Although each family member had mostly recovered from the illness, the family unit was still trying to regain its normal rhythm.

When McGruder arrived in midmorning she went right to work in the kitchen. She had found that participating in the daily chores was a much less intrusive way to observe the goings-on in the household than sitting in a corner with a notebook. Over the course of the morning she watched Amina prepare food for a dozen hungry mouths, negotiate the payment of school fees with a local official, send family members on a variety of errands, and deal with minor setbacks, including a large pot of ginger tea that had unexpectedly curdled. On top of this she did her best to keep the children (and

McGruder) from disturbing Hemed or Kimwana, both of whom were more upset that morning than usual.

In her notebook McGruder listed the stressors Amina dealt with that day. There were the relentless financial worries, three family members who needed constant care, over a dozen mouths to feed, and a small pack of children to be protected and cared for. McGruder crossed off one theory that might account for the differences in outcome of schizophrenia between developing and industrialized nations: the idea that life was simpler and less stressful for poor people living in more traditional cultures. McGruder suspects that this theory springs from a fantasy on the part of Westerners, who are soul-weary from lives of commuting, competing, and trying to find time for family. We want there to be a place in the world where our life might distill to a simple combination of satisfying work and close human interaction. In reality, a stress-free life was as elusive in Zanzibar as anywhere else in the world.

Despite the *zogozogo* and the hardships, however, Kimwana's behavior and her deficits were tolerated with remarkable equanimity. While Kimwana's activities and social interactions were often reported to McGruder as a gauge of her wellness, McGruder rarely witnessed Amina or anyone else in the family pressure Kimwana into displaying normal behaviors. During periods when Kimwana was feeling well, for instance, Amina would report that she had washed the dishes or swept the house. But Amina didn't assume a cause and an effect between productivity and wellness. This goes against some basic tenets of Western occupational therapy, which suggests that the path to mental health can be found in productivity and participation in group activity. Although the family viewed her participation in household chores as a sign of health, they didn't pressure her to perform chores with the assumption that they were curative. Indeed, when Kimwana was doing poorly, the family allowed and even encouraged her to withdraw from activity and to rest. Often, when she tried to help out during such times, her family cautioned her not to overextend herself.

For the most part, however, Kimwana was allowed to drift back and forth from illness to relative health without much monitoring or comment by the rest of the family. Periods of troubled behavior were not greeted with expressions of concern or alarm, and neither were times of wellness celebrated. As such, Kimwana felt little pressure to self-identify as someone with a permanent mental illness. This stood in contrast with the diagnosis of schizophrenia as McGruder knew it was used in the West. There the diagnosis carries the assumption of a chronic condition, one that often comes to define a person.

The prizing of rest over work and passive acceptance of abnormal behavior versus active encouragement or criticism were representative of an overall calm emotional tone in the household. Even on difficult days there was an air of tolerance when dealing with Hemed's and Kimwana's disturbed behavior. McGruder believed that this tone emanated not simply from the personalities in this particular family but from cultural cues in Zanzibar, and she took it as her mission to find the sources that created this emotionally even atmosphere.

Emotional Expression and Schizophrenia

The early research into the relationship between the emotional temperature within families and the long-term course of schizophrenia took place in England in the 1950s. Clinicians had anecdotally observed that some patients with schizophrenia released from hospital care came back within a short period of time, whereas other patients managed to stay out of inpatient care for longer periods. A team of researchers led by the psychiatrist George Brown decided to try to figure out what factors might distinguish the two groups. They conducted lengthy open-ended interviews designed to encourage first-person stories from family members. There were no right or wrong answers; researchers attempted only to elicit rich descriptions of daily life with the mentally ill family member. After categorizing all the emotional reactions they could identify, they tracked the patients over time, noting their rates of relapse and general levels of functioning.

Initially they looked at the families of the patients who fared better, but they could find no behavior that had significant predictive value. Studying the families of the high-relapse patients, however, they did find factors that appeared to predict outcomes. Three emotional reactions from family members showed a relationship with the patients with higher relapse rates. Collectively referred to as "high expressed emotion" they were criticism, hostility, and emotional overinvolvement. In particular, high-relapse patients tended to live in an environment where at least one relative routinely criticized and attempted to control the patient's behavior.*

Criticism and hostility are relatively self-explanatory. "Emotional overinvolvement," however, is a term of art that requires a little explanation. It describes a range of behaviors that may include dramatic expressions of self-sacrifice, extreme devotion, overprotectiveness, or intrusiveness in the patient's life. One mother, for

---

*Expressed emotion researchers have been careful to point out that they were not tying emotional temperatures in families to the onset of schizophrenia. High emotion was not a cause of the disease, but rather appeared to be a factor that greatly influenced its course and outcome. While there is a significant difference between families with high emotional temperatures and those with low, this is not true in every case. Many high-expressed-emotion families care for schizophrenics with low incidence of relapse, and vice versa. It should also be noted that it is not only relatives who have been studied. Similar results have come from research into high and low emotionality expressed by caretakers in group homes and mental institutions.

instance, was rated as emotionally overinvolved when she reported that she was so concerned with her son's condition that she had dropped all other interests from her life. Her sole activity, she reported, was to take care of him and protect him, "like a pearl or a diamond." This same mother said that she often became so distraught over her son's plight that she considered committing suicide by shooting herself, running out into traffic, and throwing herself down the family staircase.

Researchers have found a connection with high expressed emotion (EE) and poorer outcomes with some other mental illnesses, but nowhere is it as pronounced as with schizophrenia. Why is there such a strong connection? Researchers believe that the experience of being criticized or constantly observed and judged parallels the experience of the disease itself. It is not coincidence, in other words, that one of the central symptoms of schizophrenia is hearing demanding, critical, or disparaging voices. Social stress is a known trigger for psychotic episodes, and a number of studies testing diastolic blood pressure, skin conductance, and electrodermal reactivity all pointed to the connection between high-expressed-emotion relatives and increased feelings of stress in a patient. When confronted with relatives known for their high levels of expressed emotion, researchers could watch as dials measuring bodily stress rose in the patient.

This connection between high-expressed-emotion households and relapse rates proved true across cultures. Over the course of the 1970s and 1980s dozens of studies were conducted on populations in Denmark, Italy, Germany, Spain, France, North America (including both Anglos and Mexican Americans), China, Taiwan, India, North Africa, and Australia. In a paper that aggregated the data from a dozen studies, researchers noted that the relapse rates were *three to seven times greater* for patients from high-expressed-emotion families. The connection remained even when the severity of the initial symptoms and drug compliance were taken into account. In another paper that brought together the data from twenty-five studies, researchers found that the relapse rate was 50 percent for high-expressed-emotion families and 21 percent for low-expressed-emotion families.

God's Blessings

McGruder could sense that Amina's household had a low level of expressed emotion when it came to dealing with Hemed and Kimwana, but it took her quite a while to understand the cultural sources of that tone. She spent a good deal of her time trying to tease out the local religious beliefs that wove themselves around the ideas of madness in Zanzibar. Like 90 percent of Zanzibaris, Amina's family belonged to the Sunni Shafi'ites sect. This is an Islamic sect that believes in adhering faithfully to the teachings of the Koran and the stories collected by Al-Bukhari that recount the life of the Prophet Mohammed. It is from these stories, collectively called a hadith, that many Zanzibaris draw wisdom to manage the everyday challenges of life.

Both the Koran and Al-Bukhari's hadith recount ideas about suffering and hardship that McGruder could see had deeply informed the family's treatment of Kimwana and Hemed. Amina and other family members often repeated the belief that Allah would never put more burdens on a person than he or she could bear. "In our family we have this challenge but this is just life," Amina would tell McGruder when talking about Kimwana and Hemed. "Other people have other problems. Maybe their house has burned down. Everyone knows their own burden best."

McGruder came to understand that these were not just bromides. In the family's Muslim belief, managing hardships provided a way to pay the debt of sinfulness. Illness or bad turns of fortune were seen as neither arbitrary nor a punishment. Rather, they believed that God's grace awaited those who not only endured suffering but were grateful for the opportunity to prove their ability to endure it. In this way Amina's remarkable ability to stay steady and resolute in the presence of sick and disabled family members was an expression of her religious belief.

McGruder had heard similar "God willed it" sentiments repeated among Christians in the United States, but the embrace of hardships in Zanzibar was qualitatively different. Although American Christians might believe that God had sent a challenge or a misfortune, they were also likely to believe that God had given them the strength not just to embrace the difficulty but to overcome it or learn a valuable lesson. In the cosmology of Western Christians, life's challenges provide opportunities to become stronger and to have a closer relationship with God. The burdens God sends to Christians in the Western world are incitements to self-improvement. The comforts that Amina found in her religious belief, by contrast, were not in an encouragement to overcome or learn from hardships. Rather, simply accepting her burdens was a continuous act of penance.

"Religion as I understood it as a child had more to do with what you believed than what you did during your day," McGruder told me. "Here in Zanzibar religion has much more to do with what you do. You can see it in how people live their lives, how they pray five times a day and fast during Ramadan." In McGruder's view, the steady care given to Kimwana and especially Hemed seemed to come out of the family's religious desire to prove worthy of the burden God had given them.

Sometimes it seemed that their acceptance of burdens bordered on the fatalistic. "Fatalism" is not a word McGruder would employ, given that its negative connotations violate the anthropologist's credo to remain judgment-neutral. Still, McGruder found herself using such phrases as "acquiescence in the face of adversity" and "embracing difficulties as a natural part of life" almost as euphemisms. She remembers times when she tried not to let her jaw drop at the family's lack of upset. One such moment came when Kimwana took an overdose of her medication and ended up in the hospital. "There was no noisy woe-is-me talk or dramatic wringing of hands. They seemed to take it in stride like everything else," McGruder recalls. "When I asked what I could do, Amina told me that I could take a carton of milk to Kimwana in the hospital. So I took the milk." For McGruder, a fighter and problem solver by nature, it took some time to recognize the benefits of such acceptance of life's difficulties.

The Creatures in Our Heads

The other religious belief that was central to the family's conception of the illness was spirit possession. It would be easy for a Westerner to assume that belief in spirit possession would almost certainly increase the stigma for a mentally ill person. McGruder remembered the horror stories of spirit possession she learned as a child in the United States. Those beliefs were informed more by pop cultural representations (such as the movie *The Exorcist*) than by what she heard in church. Nevertheless her cultural understanding of these devil-focused narratives about spirit possession included dramatic suffering and ostracism for the person believed to be possessed. In the Christian context, possession is nearly always thought of as a profoundly disturbing experience, usually requiring dramatic and sometimes violent interventions. Given the choice between the biomedical understanding of schizophrenia and the spirit possession narrative, most Westerners assume the drier science-bound explanation for the disease would certainly inflame less emotion and stigma. As McGruder came to understand the spirit possession beliefs of families like Amina's, however, she found them to be very different from Christian beliefs in the West. To begin with, spirit possession in Zanzibar was not an uncommon or necessarily an extreme experience. As Amina explained to McGruder, we all have "creatures in our heads."

The beliefs surrounding spirit possession in Zanzibar arose from the complex combination of traditional Swahili culture and Arabic beliefs about *jinns*. These spirits that often inhabit living individuals aren't uniformly good or bad but can cause problems if they are not dealt with in appropriate ways. A spirit handed down from one's ancestor is generally thought to have a protective effect for the person who carries it. Such an entity will cause difficulties only if it is ignored or not properly appeased. These spirits can have an ethnicity, gender, and religious affiliation of their own. A spirit might be picked up accidentally or through witchcraft. Sorcerers are said to raise and feed spirits, which they use to harm their enemies.

The main difference between the character of spirits and of humans, McGruder learned, is that spirits are often autonomous, rude, selfish, and not given to concealing their emotions. (In this way they are sometimes compared to tourists who intrude but do not greet.) When a spirit possesses someone, he or she often violates the social norms. A sister momentarily influenced by a spirit may strike a brother who is harassing or threatening her, for instance.

Because nearly everyone on the island believed in spirit possession and had a personal experience with it, the application of the belief to mental illness had the counterintuitive effect of lessening the stigma attached to the behavior of the mentally ill person. It made bizarre or disruptive behavior more understandable and forgivable. Like the sister who has a ready explanation for hitting her brother, mentally ill persons and their family can evoke the narrative of spirit possession to explain unusual or antisocial behavior.

Belief in spirit possession also gives the family a sense of agency in that it allows for a variety of socially accepted interventions. "Spirits causing problems are not exorcised in the Christian sense of casting out demons," McGruder explains. "Rather they are coaxed with food and goods, feted with song, dance. They are placated, settled, reduced in malfeasance." It was common, for instance, to write phrases from the Koran on the inside edges of a teacup with saffron paste and then to dissolve the writing so that the ill person could literally imbibe the holy words. Similarly the Koran might be read over water before it was used for bathing. Pagan spirits would be driven away by such acts, and Muslim spirits would become subdued. Kimwana found such activities calming. She especially enjoyed it when family members read to her the short verses from the Koran that children learn to read and memorize early in school. "If someone reads and I listen, then my mind clears," Kimwana said. "It tells us to become compliant and wait patiently. I listen to the Koran and then I rest."

For McGruder the point was not that these practices were effective in combating the biological causes of schizophrenia. Rather, they were simple examples of how the spirit possession narratives kept the sick person within the social group. Importantly, the idea that spirits could come and go allowed the person with schizophrenia a cleaner bill of health when the illness went into remission. An ill individual enjoying a time of relative health could employ the spirit possession story to, at least temporarily, retake his or her responsibilities in the kinship group.

In all these ways the belief in spirit possession could decrease the sense of blame or shame carried by the family or the ill individual. The blessings and burdens of God and the mysteries of the spirit world were, after all, beyond the ability of the individual or family to effectively control. As McGruder observed, "When humans do not assume they have rather complete control of their experience, they do not so deeply fear those who appear to have lost it."

In some ways the low expressed emotional atmosphere in the family stood in contrast to McGruder's work as a Western anthropologist trying diligently to understand it. At times she had to remind herself to turn off her analytical gaze, her desire to document and categorize the behavior she was there to witness.

She remembers one day when Kimwana invited her to sit with her on the steps of the family's interior courtyard. McGruder could tell from the liveliness in her eyes that Kimwana was more fully present than she had been recently. Kimwana sat, barefoot, with her back against the door frame, and talked of how enjoyable it was to feel the breeze. McGruder asked her what she had been doing prior to her arrival that day and Kimwana told her that she had been resting but not sleeping.

"When you rest, do you think a lot?" McGruder asked.

"Yes, I think so much," Kimwana admitted.

"What do you think about?"

"For example," Kimwana answered, "just now I was thinking if I would get better."

It was a promising opening. McGruder sensed that it would be a good time to ask her more questions about her disease experience. But then she found she could not bring herself to risk breaking the peacefulness of the moment. Making the ill individual aware that his or her behavior and cognition are being monitored and judged was, she knew, a sign of emotional overinvolvement. So as much as she wanted to question Kimwana more, McGruder turned the conversation back to the quality of the breeze and how cool it was to sit in the shade of the house, trying, as best she could, not to document the low emotional intensity of the household but instead to manifest it.

Emotion across Cultures

McGruder's intent in describing Amina and her family was not to make them into heroes. Indeed what made them remarkable in her eyes was just how unremarkable they considered their sacrifice. Amina never suggested that the care she gave her crippled and mentally ill ex-husband was praiseworthy or particularly out of the ordinary. Because many other families subscribed to similar religious and cultural beliefs about the need to accept God's burdens, Amina's family's unemotional self-sacrifice was the norm in Zanzibar.

Because different cultures around the world view mental illness in different cultural contexts, the intensity of emotion attached to these experiences often varies. Researchers have found different average levels of expressed emotion not just among families but also among cultures and even among different subcultures in the same city. "To be specific," Janis Hunter Jenkins writes, "a culture provides its members with an available repertoire of affective and behavioral responses to the human condition, including illness. . . . It offers models of how people should or might feel and act in response to the serious illness of a loved one." Individuals in a given place and time will react to illness similarly, in other words, because they share the same limited repertoire of cultural scripts for how to play their part.

The different ways that cultures communicate expectations for behavior are often quite subtle. Seemingly small differences, such as the disease's name, can make a difference. Jenkins noticed, for instance, that Mexican American families in southern California, who had lower expressed emotion scores than Anglo-American families tended to use the term *nervios* to describe the illness of the relative with schizophrenia. This seemed at first an inappropriate word; *nervios* is a folk term often used as a generic way to describe any one of a whole range of symptoms, including headaches, dizziness, sleeping disorders, aggressive or grumpy behavior as well as feelings of anxiety, insecurity, or fear. *Nervios* is a catchall diagnosis for feelings of disquiet or distress. The use of the term appeared to be a kind of culturally inspired, willful blindness for these family members. Calling schizophrenia *nervios* was the equivalent of telling someone with cancer that he is just feeling under the weather.

On closer examination, though, there appeared to be a subtle purpose behind the misnomer. Jenkins saw that the use of the word was part of a strategy by which the family jointly downplayed the gravity of the illness. *Nervios* carried little of the dire connotations an Anglo-American would associate with schizophrenia. *Nervios*, like spirit possession, is thought of as a transitory state. This allowed relatives and the ill family member to regard periods of remission in a more favorable light.

This hopeful naming also fostered feelings of empathy. Many of the Mexican American family members in one of Jenkins's studies told her that they too had suffered from *nervios*, in a milder form, and so could empathize with the relative's distress. "In this way," Jenkins concluded, "conception of the illness as nervios enables the maintenance of close identification of family members by fostering the view that the relative is 'just like us only more so.'" The label and its connotations allowed family members to keep the relative within the fold.

That the very naming of the disease could have an impact on its outcome again highlights the distinction between a medical illness and a mental illness. The course of a metastasizing cancer is unlikely to be changed by how we talk about it. With schizophrenia, however, symptoms are largely expressed within the person's complex interactions with those around them. The key to the emotional tenor of those interactions lies to some extent in the words and cultural beliefs that surround the disease.

Because these words and narratives are shared by cultures, it is not surprising that the average level of expressed emotion varies from place to place. Comparing different groups around the world, it turns out that urban Anglo-Americans have the highest level of expressed emotion on average. In one study over 67 percent of Anglo-American families with a schizophrenic family member were rated as "high-EE." Of the other groups studied:

Among British families 48 percent were high EE
Among Chinese families 42 percent
Among American families of Mexican descent 41 percent
Among British Sikh families 30 percent
Among Indian families 23 percent

What does it mean that European American families have the highest average levels of expressed emotion? Is this an indication that white Americans lack the sympathy or the kindness to care for their mentally ill?

Professor Jill Hooley of Harvard University conducted a study to understand what distinguishes high-EE relatives from their less emotionally intense counterparts. She gave both high- and low-EE relatives a simple test that measures what psychologists call "locus of control." Basically she wanted to know to what extent these relatives believed they had individual control over their own lives. To determine this she asked them whether they agreed or disagreed with statements such as the following:

- When I make plans, I am almost certain that I can make them work.

- I believe a person really can be a master of his fate.

- I can control my own problems only if I have outside support.

- A great deal of what happens to me is probably a matter of luck.

Those who tended to agree with statements such as the first two were thought to have an internal locus of control. They were the type of people who thought of themselves as captains of their own destiny, able to shape their future through force of will. Those who agreed with statements similar to the second two were thought to have an external locus of control, meaning they believed that the course of their lives was largely influenced by factors outside themselves.

Hooley found that relatives who were highly critical of the mentally ill family members were those with an internal locus of control. Their critical comments to the mentally ill person didn't mean that they were cruel or uncaring; they were simply applying to their relative the same assumptions about human nature that they applied to themselves. "An internal based locus of control reflects an approach to the world that is active, resourceful, and that emphasizes personal accountability," concluded Hooley. "Thus, far from high criticism reflecting something negative about the family members of patients with schizophrenia, high criticism (and hence high EE) was associated with a characteristic that is widely regarded as positive."

Widely regarded as positive, that is, in the United States. It has long been noted that countries and cultures differ in their shared beliefs about locus of control and related measures such as scales of individualism versus collectivism or egocentric versus sociocentric conceptions of self. In many cross-cultural studies, the cliché that Americans are more individualistic proves to be true. In a masterful meta-analysis of dozens of cross-cultural studies performed over the past fifty years, professor of psychology Daphna Oyserman and colleagues from the University of Michigan concluded that, compared with other groups around the world, European Americans are indeed "more individualistic—valuing personal independence more. . . . To contemporary Americans, being an individualist is not only a good thing; it is a quintessentially American thing."

Viewed in the most positive light, these highly emotionally involved relatives were more hopeful about the disease because they remained convinced that the ill family member should be able to overcome the symptoms with an application of personal will. "It is plausible to speculate," Hooley and a colleague in another paper on the topic concluded, "that certain cultural values (e.g., fatalism) in traditional groups might engender more benign and less blaming attributions toward those with mental illnesses. In contrast, cultural values that emphasize individuality, achievement, and personal accountability might be expected to facilitate more attributions of responsibility and control in the context of disturbed behavior."

In his book *Crazy: A Father's Search through America's Mental Health Madness,* Pete Earley vividly documents a common response among Western parents when faced with the onset of a severe mental illness in their child. One typical father described his reaction to the schizophrenic break of his son: "I went to the library and began reading books about mental illness. . . . I thought: 'No, I'm going to fix this.' That is your first instinct as a parent. You're going to fix it. I thought, 'I can get him help. I can get him cured.'" This intense can-do spirit is admirable and often heartbreaking. Because there is no silver bullet cure for schizophrenia, families who attack the problem looking to fix it are often frustrated by the results. That intense focus, even when it springs from a hopeful engagement of the problem, might be the very thing that exacerbates the illness.

"Mental illness is feared and has such a stigma because it represents a reversal of what Western humans have come to value as the essence of human nature," McGruder believes. "Because our culture so highly values self-control and control of circumstances, we become abject when contemplating mentation that seems more changeable, less restrained and less controllable, more open to outside influence, than we imagine our own to be."

When the Biomedical Narrative Comes to Town

All of the patients with schizophrenia that McGruder interviewed in Zanzibar received at least some treatment from doctors trained in other countries. During the country's communist years, foreign doctors came from East Germany and China. More recently they hail from the United States and Britain. Over that time chronically mentally ill patients in Zanzibar were prescribed a wide range of the psychopharmacological drugs that are now ubiquitous around the world.

During the years that McGruder studied mental illness in Zanzibar, she watched as traditional beliefs began to mix with biomedical explanations of mental illness. For some families, such as Amina's, those two understandings didn't necessarily compete with each other. The idea that spirit possession was causing bizarre behavior coexisted with the notion that the pills from the doctors might help her daughter's quality of life. One does not have to believe the "brain disease" explanation, after all, to take a pill.

In some families that McGruder studied, however, the introduction of Western ideas about schizophrenia had a more complicated and problematic effect.

Shazrin al-Mitende was 43 when McGruder began visiting her family. She lived with five adult relatives and ten children, one of whom was developmentally disabled. Shazrin's half-brother, Abdulridha, was her main caretaker, devoting much of his life to the task. The male nurse who suggested Shazrin and her family for inclusion in McGruder's study thought of Abdulridha as an excellent caretaker.

Abdulridha himself certainly agreed with this assessment. In their first meeting he listed for McGruder all the ways that he had taken charge of his sister's life. "It is necessary that I give up my own activities so much in order to care for her," he said. At another point he told McGruder, "I am like her slave now. She says 'bring me some water.' I go and fetch it. It is she who should be bringing me water."

As McGruder got to know the family, she learned Shazrin's history. Trouble began in 1968, when Shazrin was just 13, on the night of the new moon that signals the end of Ramadan. Shazrin was sitting with a group of women relatives applying henna designs to each other's hands. This group beautification was in preparation for the feasting and gathering of relatives that followed the end of the month-long daylight fast. As she sat with the other women, the sight of a black cat walking through the room startled her. During the feasting the next day, she told her family that she felt unwell and overheated. When her mother told her to lie down and tried to help her out of her new dress, Shazrin began to scream uncontrollably. She was inconsolable for several days.

Because her behavior could be traced to the sighting of the black cat, it was at first agreed that spirit possession was behind her strange and disruptive behavior. Shazrin's grandfather had been a spirit cult practitioner, who, it was said, conjured spirits in the family courtyard. Some family members and neighbors assumed that one of those spirits, set free of the grandfather's control at his death, had alighted on the soul of Shazrin.

Shazrin's family took her to see several traditional doctors. They traveled up and down the Swahili Coast consulting with healers in Dar es Salaam, Bagamoyo, and Tanga in Tanzania and traveling as far away as Mombasa in Kenya. In one instance her hair was shaved and small cuts were made in her scalp into which herbal medicines were rubbed. Other healers used techniques intended to call forth the spirit so it could be negotiated with and placated. Another healer was skilled in diagnosing ailments by drawing pictures of the patient. Despite these efforts, Shazrin improved little.

As it happened, a young neighbor had recently become a doctor at the local mental hospital. He persuaded the family that Shazrin should be taken to Kidongo Chekundu Mental Hospital the next time her behavior became difficult to control. And so, when Shazrin became disturbed a few weeks later, the family called the police, who took her to be admitted. She was still only 13 years old, a frightened girl in a locked ward for adults with severe mental illnesses. In those first hospital records, the staff noted that she was restless and preoccupied but mostly rational.

It was during this time that she briefly came under the care of an American psychiatrist named Charles Swift, who was having a dramatic impact on Tanzania's evolving treatment of the mentally ill. He had come to the newly formed country in 1966 intending to stay only two years but ended up staying eight, working mostly in hospitals on the mainland. From the perspective of Tanzania's Ministry of Health, Swift was a godsend. When he arrived he was the only trained psychiatrist in the country.

Once a month Swift would fly from Dar es Salaam to Zanzibar and visit the mental hospital, where the medical director put him to work diagnosing difficult cases. One of those patients was the young Shazrin. She remembers being frightened in the presence of this American. "He was very fierce," she says. It was Swift who first diagnosed her condition as schizophrenia.

Shazrin's assessment of Swift as "fierce" stands in sharp contrast to the caring and rather humble man he presents to the reader in *Dar Days,* his memoir of his time in Tanzania. He reports having disdained the superior attitude of the former British colonialists he met in the country. But while it is clear that Swift took pains to be culturally sensitive, he also had a great certainty in the value of the expertise he brought to the country. He clearly saw his service as parallel to medical doctors who brought state-of-the-art practices and medication to places where local clinicians had little knowledge or resources to battle disease.

Humble as he may have been, he did not turn down the status he was granted as a mental health professional from the Western world. Looking back at Swift's tenure in Tanzania, it is not surprising that he extended his stay by six years. Back in New Jersey he worked for a medium-size child development center, but in Tanzania he was a central player in establishing the mental health system for the entire country. His advice was sought in every aspect of the country's approach to mental illness, and he dined regularly with politicians and dignitaries.

In his memoir Swift makes it clear that the pervasive beliefs in spirits and witchcraft were a problem for the population. Replacing such native beliefs with clear and unemotional Western diagnoses seemed to him an obvious improvement. It was Swift's hope that by providing Western knowledge he could help erase these myths that he believed brought stigma to the mentally ill. For Shazrin, his diagnosis would have long-lasting effects.

For the next two decades Shazrin was in and out of the mental hospital dozens of times, for both long and short stays. Overall she spent nearly one-fifth of her young adulthood at Chekundu. Her records show that she took a variety of medications during that period, including, for a time, a large fifty-milligram dose of the antipsychotic fluphenazine every two weeks. During another period the doctors prescribed her a nightly dose of the barbiturate sodium amytal. In the late 1970s she also underwent a series of electroconvulsive treatments. Some of the medication brought on epileptic-like fits and made her lips and hands tremble uncontrollably.

Shazrin's treatment at the hospital wasn't the only way that Western medicine affected her life. Over the course of her illness her half-brother, Abdulridha, increasingly distanced himself from the beliefs of traditional healers and aligned himself more and more with Western notions and treatments of his sister's condition. He associated Western medicine and Western beliefs about mental illness with his self-conception of being a modern and educated man.

Abdulridha acquired his knowledge about Western understandings of mental illness from a variety of sources. He learned much from the doctors at the hospital. Of all the family members McGruder interviewed, Abdulridha was the only one who understood the distinction between the symptoms of schizophrenia and the side effects, including tremors and weight gain, of the antipsychotic medication. He was also the only one to understand that some of Shazrim's medications were taken to control the side effects of other drugs.

He picked up information from other sources as well. For instance, from a Voice of America program about drugs that treat depression he came to the conclusion that Western doctors had a medicine that would cure his sister's uncontrollable bouts of crying. As understood by Abdulridha, the biomedical approach implied that his sister's mind was broken but fixable through medication.

McGruder began to think that she was watching a classic display of emotional overinvolvement as she observed Abdulridha attempt to manage every aspect of his sister's existence. What particularly intrigued McGruder was how Abdulridha used his biomedical orientation toward the disease to justify his control over Shazrin. Aligning himself with the Western doctors, he allowed himself to express intense frustration at his sister for her apparently stubborn refusal to get better. Shazrin's lack of recovery despite his efforts and those of the doctors appeared to embarrass and infuriate him. "I tell her, 'I do everything for you,'" he recounted to McGruder. "'You should stop all those behaviors in order to give me some encouragement.'"

McGruder had a front-row seat in witnessing how the biomedical explanation affected Abdulridha's treatment of his sister. She was even, at times, recruited against her will into the dynamic. For Abdulridha, McGruder was a representative of modern Western knowledge and authority, and he attempted to co-opt her presence in the life of the family to prove that his opinions and actions were backed up by doctors and educated people.

When McGruder came to visit, Abdulridha took pride in reciting for her every detail of Shazrin's daily activities. He was particularly forthcoming about his knowledge of her menstrual cycle, detailing the precise dates menses began and ended. He would then tell her of any recent bad behavior. "She has finished bleeding some three days ago now, but her condition is still bad," he said in one typical encounter. That he openly talked about such aspects of Shazrin's life startled McGruder. A brother talking about such things was a clear violation of the rules of modesty she had observed elsewhere in Zanzibar. Abdulridha's biomedical conception of his sister's illness appeared to invalidate normal rules of conduct. Similarly he would often talk about Shazrin as if she could not hear him. At these times she would go blank and stare at the floor, refusing to respond to anyone. "This is the problem," Abdulridha said at one point when his sister's affect went flat. "She is not here at all now; she has been completely covered. I told you you would see it."

Needless to say, being forced into an alliance that excluded Shazrin was uncomfortable for McGruder; she worried that her presence was actually helping Abdulridha stigmatize his sister. In her field notes she wrote, "I am finding it progressively harder to write about this family and harder still to visit them. The events . . . have convinced me that family interactions definitely increase Shazrin's suffering and I am now included against my will in that process."

In the end Abdulridha's increasing alliance with Western medicine had the effect of stripping away the local beliefs held by other families McGruder had studied in Zanzibar. Unlike Kimwana's family, there was no safe harbor in the belief that God had sent the illness as a blessing, a burden to be embraced. Those beliefs were replaced by a set of ideas that appeared to allow Abdulridha to dehumanize his sister and justify his harsh control over her life.

The Rise of the Biomedical Narrative in the West

Over the past two generations, Western psychologists and psychiatrists have promoted the biomedical approach to mental illness around the world with the argument that adopting this way of thinking would lessen the stigma surrounding these conditions. Even patient and family advocacy groups such as the National Alliance for the Mentally Ill in the United States and SANE in the United Kingdom have consistently promoted the idea that mental illnesses should be viewed as medical illnesses, as "diseases of the brain."

Western mental health professionals coined the term "mental health literacy" to describe the set of ideas they've promoted around the world. Populations are considered more "literate" if they adopt Western biomedical conceptions of these diseases. A study from the World Psychiatric Association, for instance, identified respondents as "knowledgeable" and "sophisticated" when they identified schizophrenia as a "debilitating disease." Another study portrayed those who endorsed the statement that "mental illness is an illness like any other" as having a "knowledgeable, benevolent, supportive orientation towards the mentally ill."

The logic seemed unassailable: once people believed that the symptoms of mental illnesses such as schizophrenia were not the choice of the individual and did not spring from supernatural forces, the sufferer would be protected from blame. The brain disease narrative would make it less likely that the public would attribute the onset of mental illness to an individual's life choices or a weakness of character. In addition, people would be less likely to connect the difficulty of recovery to a patient's lack of personal will or motivation. By pushing the blame onto the functioning of genes or broken biochemistry in the brain, the individual could escape stigma.

Studies show that over the past fifty years the world has steadily adopted this medical model of mental illness. Although these changes have happened most dramatically in the United States and Europe, similar shifts have been documented around the world. When asked to name the sources of mental illness, people from every country studied are increasingly likely to mention "chemical imbalance" or "brain disease" or "genetics" as part of the cause of mental illness. These global changes in belief represent a hard-won victory on the part of mental health care providers, drug companies, and advocacy organizations.

Unfortunately, as mental health professionals and advocates for the mentally ill have been winning this rhetorical and conceptual battle, they've been simultaneously losing the war against stigma. Studies of attitudes in the United States between the 1950s and 1996 have demonstrated that the perception of dangerousness surrounding the mentally ill has steadily *increased* over this time. Similarly a study in Germany found that the public's desire to maintain distance from those diagnosed with schizophrenia increased between 1990 and 2001.

Researchers hoping to figure out what was causing this rise in stigma found a startling connection. It turns out that those who adopted the biomedical and genetic beliefs about mental illness were most often those who wanted less contact with the mentally ill or thought of them as dangerous and unpredictable. This unfortunate cause-and-effect relationship has held up in numerous studies around the world. In a study conducted in Turkey, for example, those who labeled schizophrenic behavior as *akil hastaligi* (illness of the brain or reasoning abilities) were more inclined to assert that schizophrenics were aggressive and should not live free in the community than those who saw the disorder as *ruhsal hastagi* (a disorder of the spiritual or inner self). Another study, which looked at populations in Germany, Russia, and Mongolia, found that "irrespective of place . . . endorsing biological factors as the cause of schizophrenia was associated with a greater desire for social distance." The authors of that study concluded that "promulgating biological concepts among the public might not contribute to a desired reduction in social distance towards people with mental disorders."

The problem, it appears, is that the biomedical or genetic narrative about an illness such as schizophrenia carries with it the subtle assumption that a brain made ill through biomedical or genetic abnormalities is more thoroughly broken and permanently abnormal compared to one made ill though life events. "Genetic arguments may work in an asymmetric fashion," wrote researcher Jason Schnittker from the University of Pennsylvania. "They encourage the view that mental illness is impersonal and uncontrollable in its development, but more stable and unyielding in its course. By the same token genetic arguments inflate perception of dangerousness in so far as [they imply that] the mentally ill are always at risk for violence even when treated. . . . Genetic arguments make the person appear even more 'at risk' and threatening."

In a dramatic experiment, Professor Sheila Mehta from Auburn

University in Montgomery, Alabama, effectively answered the question of how these beliefs about mental illness can translate into behaviors between people. In her study, subjects were led to understand that they were participating in a simple learning task with a partner, who was actually a confederate in the study. Before the experiment started, the two partners exchanged some biographical data, during which the confederate told the test subject that he suffered from a mental illness. Confederates then stated either "[The illness occurred due to] some things that happened to me as a kid" (the psychosocial explanation) or "I had a disease just like any other which affected my biochemistry" (the disease explanation). The learning experiment called for the test subject to supposedly teach the confederate a certain pattern of button presses. The only feedback the test subject could give to incorrect button pushes was a mild to "somewhat painful" electrical shock.

Analyzing the data, Mehta found a dramatic difference between the group of subjects given the psychosocial explanation for their partner's mental illness history and those given the brain disease explanation. Those who believed that their partner suffered an "illness like any other" increased the severity of the shocks at a faster rate than those who believed they were partnered with someone who had a mental disorder caused by childhood events. Mehta concluded, "The result of the study suggests that we may actually treat people more harshly when their problem is described in disease terms. . . . We say we are being kind but our actions suggest otherwise. . . . The disease view engenders a less favorable estimation of the mentally disordered than the psychosocial view." She added, "Viewing those with mental disorders as diseased sets them apart and may lead to our perceiving them as physically distinct. Biochemical aberrations make them almost a different species."

Indeed it was just this dynamic that McGruder witnessed between Shazrin and her brother. Remarkably, despite more than forty years of evidence suggesting that the biomedical or brain disease belief increases stigma, the Western mental health professionals continue to promote these ideas with vigor.

Just Chemistry

One afternoon McGruder took me to the Kidongo Chekundu Mental Hospital, a few miles from downtown Stone Town. The compound was made up of several single-story white stucco structures with tiled roofs surrounding a large courtyard. There was an intake area where patients and their families sat on benches waiting to be seen, a documents room, and an area where meals were prepared over a wood fire. McGruder showed me the occupational therapy room she had helped establish many years ago. Hundreds of paintings and drawings by former patients hung on the wall.

The facility for housing the patients was separated into an open ward for patients considered to be of no danger to themselves or others and two locked areas for the women and men who were more seriously disturbed. In the courtyard I talked with a young man who was lighting a small cooking fire to boil water for tea. His English was perfect, with an American accent. I assumed he was a doctor or a caretaker until he told me he had come from the mainland for a long stay at the hospital while the doctors attempted to find the right balance of medication for his manic depression. He was excited to talk to me. He had gone to college in Arizona and had fond memories of the States.

Later two guards led me to the entryway of the locked area of the men's compound. For a few minutes several men on the other side of a barred window talked animatedly at me in Kiswahili. Behind them I could see a half dozen other men in the open area. Some were sleeping, and others rocked restlessly.

Given my cultural background, I was incapable of believing that these men were possessed by spirits. Indeed I find it difficult to think of the biological explanation for mental illness as fungible cultural "belief" or "narrative." I assume, in short, that it is the scientific truth. But as I later thought of my brief visit to the locked ward at Kidongo Chekundu I began to wonder about the meaning behind these certainties.

If you ask me what it means that schizophrenia is related to genes, for instance, I will say that people with a family history of schizophrenia are at greater risk. Although this appears to be statistically true, that is pretty much the extent of my actual knowledge on the topic of the genetic precursors to schizophrenia. My scientific understanding of abnormalities in brain chemistry related to the disease is similarly limited. So although I deeply believe that the biomedical explanation for mental illness is likely true, that certainty does not come with a degree in biochemistry or genetics.

If these beliefs have so little weight, why do I continue to hold to them so tightly? Beliefs about mental illness—and this is as true in the United States as it is in Zanzibar—are first and foremost testaments to group membership. By attesting to my biomedical orientation, I am placing myself in that group of people who I believe have a "sophisticated" and "knowledgeable" orientation to the mentally ill. I am placing myself in the group of doctors, biomedical researchers, clinicians, and scientists. Note that, unlike the spirit possession belief common in Zanzibar, the group I'm affiliating myself with does not include the mentally ill themselves.

Aside from their objective truth or falsehood, one meaningful way to compare cultural beliefs about mental illness is to ask this simple question: Which cultural beliefs tend to exclude the sufferer from the social group and which allow the ill individual to remain part of the group?

Accounts written by patients themselves and their loved ones make it clear just how stigmatizing the biomedical explanation can be. Here, for example, is D. A. Granger writing of his experiences years after being diagnosed with schizophrenia in his first year of Harvard Medical School:

> I have spent years . . . clinging to the understanding that I was a defective biological unit. . . . This may truly be a valuable perspective for those who observe mental illness, but for me, as a subject, this tree bore only dry and tasteless fruit. . . .
>
> > I have a chemical imbalance; I really didn't feel those things.
> > I have a chemical imbalance; I didn't really experience those things.
> > I have a chemical imbalance; I didn't really think those things . . .
>
> Here is an insight! The entire human drama of love, suffering, ecstasy, and joy, just chemistry.

Jay Neugeboren, writing about his schizophrenic brother, similarly asked, "[If he] . . . doesn't hold onto his illness and its history as a legitimate, real and unique part of his ongoing self—what of him, at fifty-two years old, will be left?"

We ask people diagnosed with schizophrenia and those who love and care for them to adopt the brain chemistry narrative without consideration of the cost: the devaluing of the perceptions that make up the ill individual's very sense of self. Indeed, as Granger suggests, the fact that healthy people do not dwell on the "brain chemistry" story as an explanation for their own moods and feelings should be an indication of how unappealing and dehumanizing the idea is. When we fall in love, get jealous, feel the joy of playing with a child, or experience religious ecstasy we do not describe the experience to friends as a fortunate or unfortunate confluence of brain chemicals. Yet we continue to suggest that the narrative of brain chemistry will be useful in lessening the stigma associated with a mentally ill person. What could be more stigmatizing than to reduce a person's perceptions and beliefs to the notion that they are "just chemistry"? It is a narrative that often pushes the ill individual outside the group, allowing those who remain in the social circle to, as Mehta observed, view the ill person as "almost a different species."

What We Can and Can't Learn

I asked McGruder on several occasions what we might learn from her research on schizophrenia in Zanzibar. She offered various possible lessons, the most obvious being a cautionary one. Simply put, we might reconsider our interventions in the parts of the world that appear to have better outcomes than we can manage in the industrialized world.

But coming away with only that warning was unsatisfying. It is part of my American character that I'm not much interested in being told what not to do. Like those highly emotionally involved caretakers, I'm interested in how to fix the problem. I wanted a positive take-away message, some recommendation for action or change. So I kept pestering McGruder, trying to get her to be prescriptive. What had she learned from her Zanzibari research that we might be able to use in the United States to help the mentally ill?

One late afternoon, a week into my visit to Zanzibar, McGruder and I were sitting in her small apartment in Stone Town waiting for Kassim to get back from the final day of mourning his daughter. McGruder was folding laundry. By this point in the trip we had an easy rapport, although I was feeling like a houseguest who had overstayed. I turned on my tape recorder and again quizzed her on what we might learn from the way the locals address and deal with serious mental illness. Instead of answering the question on a theoretical level, this time she told me a story.

After she and her former husband, an African American whom I'll call Ed, returned from her year of research in Zanzibar they had difficulty settling back into their American lives. McGruder was back teaching and trying to bang out her dissertation. Their marriage was in a rough patch and they fought about money.

Ed, McGruder told me, had been discontent since returning from Africa. He tried out a couple of different businesses but struggled to get them off the ground. At some point he got hooked up with an aggressive multilevel financial marketing group. He went to seminars that were like revival meetings, where motivational speakers told the attendees that they could achieve financial success by selling the company's life insurance and recruiting others into the business. McGruder sensed it was a shady outfit—their promises were too good to be true—but she deeply wanted her husband to find success and happiness. At the same time Ed started a janitorial business. With McGruder's help he bought a van and cleaning supplies and he landed some contracts with area restaurants. "He was running full speed, night and day," McGruder told me. "At the same time we were going ever further into debt because we were throwing money at the startup costs of the businesses."

Around this time McGruder went to a conference in Philadelphia. While she was away she had trouble getting Ed on the phone, which was unusual. When she landed at Sea-Tac, he came to the airport to pick her up and they went out to dinner. Ed didn't say much at dinner and seemed to be in an unusually somber mood. When they got home McGruder came down with something like food poisoning. Looking back, she wonders whether her body was picking up on something her mind couldn't yet accept.

The next morning Ed told her that he was going out. She said she was going to stay in bed and try to get some rest. Hours went by and he didn't return. At one that afternoon the police called and informed her that her husband's car had been abandoned on a local street with the motor running and doors opened.

Fearing that he had been the victim of a robbery, McGruder immediately got on the phone and called some friends for help. After retrieving the car, she called the hospitals and police stations, asking if there were any reports of injured people. It was more than twenty-four hours before they discovered that Ed had been arrested and had spent the night in the Pierce County Jail howling incoherently and ripping his clothes to shreds.

McGruder later pieced together the missing hours. After abandoning the car, Ed had jogged down the middle of a busy street. After that he switched to the railroad tracks, walking more than ten miles to the nearby town of Lakewood. Once there he entered someone's backyard, climbed into the bed of a pickup, and started throwing the contents all over the lawn. "These are the kinds of things people do when they have mania of psychotic proportions," McGruder told me. "They just don't make any sense and they can't explain to you why it seemed like a good idea at the time."

It took a full day to find Ed in the legal system because he had thrown away his identification and when asked his name would only say, "They call me Mr. Edwards." McGruder immediately understood this. "Mr. Edwards" was the name he was called by friends and neighbors during their stay in Zanzibar.

Once she found him, McGruder spent the rest of the day figuring out how to get him out on bail. After finishing the paperwork, she was told to go home and wait for a phone call, which she did. Late that afternoon her husband showed up at the door. He had been released, but no one had called her to pick him up. He had walked miles in freezing rain in nothing but a jail-issued jumpsuit.

She put him in a warm bath, where he rocked back and forth alternately crying and laughing. She tried to calm him and get him to sleep but he was restless and confused. She stayed up with him as late as she could but finally fell asleep herself. She woke to find Ed on a rampage. He had pulled out several saplings in the backyard and was in the middle of knocking everything off shelves in the kitchen and living room.

She called friends to come over and help calm Ed down and keep him from tearing apart the rest of the house. They tried to convince him that he needed to see a doctor, but he didn't seem to comprehend what they were saying. At times he would go blank; at other times he would howl and make animal noises. Finally the friends distracted Ed while McGruder called for help.

Having taught many classes on mental health and the law, McGruder believed she knew the system she was entering. She understood, for instance, that in order for Ed to be put in the hospital against his will she had to attest that he posed a danger to people or property. That part of the process turned out to be easy, and Ed was admitted into Puget Sound Hospital. Knowing what to say to get him out proved to be the hard part.

The next day McGruder went to the hospital. It was a rundown place. (It would soon be shut down by the Health Department for multiple violations, including chronic overcrowding, sexual assault in the mental wards, and dead bugs and mouse droppings in a supposedly sterile supply room.) Like many acute psychotic manias, Ed's suddenly ebbed. He was now calm and spoke rationally, telling McGruder that he was afraid to stay in the hospital. He said he was ready to go home and start seeing a doctor for his illness. McGruder was certain he had a better chance of regaining his balance if she could manage his behavior outside the hospital. She thought, "Okay, let's get him out of this place."

But the system she had triggered was not ready to let him go.

Over the next two weeks she struggled with doctors, lawyers, and judges. The first doctor she met with wanted to start Ed on five different psychiatric medications at once. McGruder knew that he could be helped by medication but argued for a more conservative approach. She was particularly put off by the judge at the commitment hearing, who appeared to be making assumptions based on Ed's race. "Has a toxicology screen been done on this man?" he asked repeatedly, even though there was no indication that the mania had been drug-induced.

Her reaction to the crisis couldn't have been more distinct from Amina's passive acceptance. McGruder was a passionate advocate for her husband at every turn. She could tell that she annoyed many of the doctors, lawyers, nurses, and clerks she interacted with. "They treated me like a nuisance for the most part," she remembers. "They treated me like I was emotionally overinvolved."

In the end, the insights she had gained while studying mental illness in Zanzibar were of little help. She was back in her own culture, and many of the Zanzibari beliefs and practices she had witnessed and so carefully documented simply didn't apply. This was true down to the level of simple logistics. McGruder and her husband lived alone and had no close kinship groups on which they could rely. They had devoted friends, but those friends all had jobs and other commitments and most lived dozens of miles away; they couldn't be counted on to care for or watch over Ed for significant periods of time. McGruder and her husband were, for the most part, alone with their burden.

McGruder did try one gambit. Ed had once been a religious man, and he began to believe that his psychotic break might have been part of God's plan. Perhaps, he suggested, God had caused the psychotic break because He wanted McGruder to better understand mental illness. "I thought that that was a little egocentric to believe that God up in heaven decided, 'She needs a little more insight,'" McGruder recalled. "But I said okay, if Ed thinks it's helpful for us to consider this possibility, I'm cool with that. That is useful. My experience in Zanzibar helped me avoid saying 'That's a crock of shit.'"

She offered to start going to church with Ed, but the religious narrative she tried to help create was an ineffective balm. Religion is a difficult palliative to employ on an as-needed basis. It either exists in one's life and surrounding culture, shaping one's conception of the self, or it does not. For Amina and her family, religion and spiritual belief permeated their lives in the same way the Koranic chants of the schoolchildren washed over their household. McGruder and her husband had no such ambient, pervasive faith to rely on, and, not surprisingly, the Christian beliefs McGruder and her husband belatedly tried to adopt proved to be of little comfort.

Try as she might, McGruder couldn't mimic the calm acquiescence Amina managed. Instead she found herself constantly monitoring Ed's behavior for signs of his mental illness. When he left the cap off the toothpaste, she found herself wondering, "Is he unable to put the cap back on because his mind is running too fast?" She began to reconsider their whole life together. She second-guessed her fond memories from their first years of dating. Had he been so charming and fun to be with because he was prone to mania? In the end the marriage failed under the pressure of Ed's illness. "Once you start looking at a loved one through the lens of a Western psychiatric diagnosis," McGruder said, "it is really hard to stop."

When McGruder finished telling me this story she was sitting on the daybed in the living room in complete darkness. The sun sets fast near the Equator, and the electricity had been out on the entire island for over a week. The air was hot and still. We sat for a time listening to the sound of footsteps echo up from the stone alleyways outside the apartment window.

"The Hallmark movie ending would be that I had learned something about mental illness in Zanzibar that I was able to use in my own time of crisis," McGruder said. "But stories of mental illness don't often have Hallmark endings."

The Transliteration

After traveling back to the United States, I kept in touch with McGruder by email. Every so often I would ask after her partner, Kassim, to see how he was dealing with the loss of his daughter. McGruder admitted in this correspondence that she herself was still trying to figure out what was going on inside his head. Despite everything she knew about different emotional expressions between cultures, she couldn't help but be concerned about his emotional flatness in the days after his daughter's death.

McGruder told me that a few days after the funeral she overheard a phone call Kassim received from a relative who had just heard about the death and wanted to travel from mainland Tanzania to offer her condolences. McGruder listened as he told the relative "Tumeshapao," meaning "We have already cooled down" or "We have healed, we are okay." When he hung up the phone, McGruder felt compelled to ask him if he really had already healed. Unable to read his outward emotions, she wanted to know whether he felt he was still grieving. She had not witnessed him weep over his daughter's death.

He explained that in the phone call he was only trying to save the relative the cost and trouble of traveling to the island. He told McGruder that he thought of his daughter often but was comforted by the fact that he had performed all of the religiously required rituals after her passing. Her body had been properly wrapped in a winding cloth and sewn into a flexible reed mat. He had carried her to the cemetery and had gotten down into the grave and arranged her body so that she was lying on her side, facing Mecca.

Later, in a different conversation, he told McGruder that since his daughter's death he had been unaccountably waking in the middle of the night, at about the time he got the telephone call, and had trouble getting back to sleep. When he finally did sleep again he was assaulted with vivid and disturbing dreams.

McGruder wondered whether his unexpressed grief was souring into depression. Kassim had a different explanation. He believed he had picked up some troubling spirits while at the graveyard burying his daughter. A few days later he went to a Koran school and paid a small fee to have a group of boys sing some Arabic prayers to the soul of his daughter. The teacher at the Koran school gave him a transliteration of the prayers so that he could pronounce the Arabic words in Kiswahili. After that, every night he recited the prayer in words he could not understand and slept soundly.

4

The Mega-Marketing of Depression in Japan

One of the chilling things about these events, whether a puzzle or a scandal, is how a very few people in key positions can determine the course of events and shape the consciousness of a generation.

DAVID HEALY

I went to visit Dr. Laurence Kirmayer in his book-lined office at McGill University in Montreal because he had a particularly good story to tell. I'd heard that a few years ago, Kirmayer had a personal brush with the pharmaceutical giant GlaxoSmithKline and the remarkable resources that the company employed to create a market for their antidepressant pill Paxil in Japan.

In person Kirmayer is the picture of a tweedy academic. He speaks in complete paragraphs in a deep authoritative voice. He has a large head and a broad face that is covered nearly to the cheekbones in a thick light-gray beard. His slightly wandering left eye suits his demeanor. If you look at the left side of his face his expression is attentive and focused on the conversation. If you look at the right side of his face he appears to be looking past you into the middle distance, as if searching for a word or pondering a thought.

In telling his story of being feted by GlaxoSmithKline, Kirmayer likes to point out that he is unaccustomed to the trappings of great wealth. Not that he's doing badly. As the director of the Division of Social and Transcultural Psychiatry at McGill, he makes a respectable living and adds to his income with a private psychiatric practice. As editor in chief of the journal *Transcultural Psychiatry,* he is well known in certain circles and can draw a crowd of admiring grad students and colleagues at an anthropology or mental health conference. But to get to those conferences he flies coach.

It was in the fall of 2000, as he tells it, that he came to understand just how *un*spectacularly rich he was. That was when he accepted an invitation from something called the International Consensus Group on Depression and Anxiety to attend two all-expenses-paid conferences, the first in Kyoto and the second a few months later on the shores of Bali.

Accepting the invitation didn't at first seem like a difficult decision. Although he knew that the conference was sponsored by an educational grant from the drug maker GlaxoSmithKline,* such industry funding wasn't unusual for academic conferences in the field of psychiatry. When he checked out the list of other invitees, he recognized all the names. It was an extremely exclusive group of highly influential clinicians and researchers from France, the United States, and Japan, among other countries. The topic, "Transcultural Issues in Depression and Anxiety," was right up his alley. Even better, he had an eager young graduate student named Junko Kitanaka who was in Japan finishing her dissertation on the history of depression in the country; such a gathering of luminaries would be a boon to her research. In addition to those

---

*Although headquartered in the UK, GlaxoSmithKline has much of its operations in the United States, where its consumer products division is based. The United States is the single largest market for GSK drugs.

incentives, attendees would be given the chance to publish their presentations in a supplement of the prestigious *Journal of Clinical Psychiatry.* "I wouldn't say it was a no-brainer, but it wasn't very hard for me to say yes," Kirmayer remembers. "How much trouble could I get in?"

His first inkling that this wasn't a run-of-the-mill academic conference came when the airline ticket arrived in the mail. This ticket was for a seat in the front of the plane and cost nearly $10,000. The next hint came when one of the conference organizers told him in no uncertain terms that these would be closed-door meetings. His grad student, Kitanaka, would not be allowed to attend. There would be no uninvited colleagues and no press.

On arrival in Kyoto in early October 2000 he found the luxury of the accommodations to be beyond anything he had personally experienced. He was ushered into an exclusive part of the hotel, where he was given a drink while an attractive woman filled out the hotel forms. His room was a palatial suite. The bath was drawn and strewn with rose petals and dosed with frangipani oil. There was a platter on the credenza filled with fruits so exotic that he could identify only the mangosteens.

"This was Gordon Gekko treatment—the most deluxe circumstances I have ever experienced in my life," Kirmayer says, smiling at the memory. This was how the other half lived, he realized—or, rather, how the other .01 percent lived. "The luxury was so far beyond anything that I could personally afford, it was a little scary. It didn't take me long to think that something strange was going on here. I wondered: What did I do to deserve this?"

Kirmayer was well aware that drug companies routinely sponsor professional conferences and educational seminars and that these events do double duty as marketing seminars. It was also common knowledge that drug makers use enticements to encourage both researchers and practitioners to attend. A prescribing doctor might be treated to a round of golf or a fancy dinner in exchange for attending an hour-long seminar about the effectiveness of some new drug. These practices are the medical equivalent of what real estate agents do to sell vacation timeshares.

But it was clear from the start that the gatherings of the International Consensus Group on Depression and Anxiety were different from the normal drug company dog and pony show, and not simply because the enticements being offered were so dear. Once the group of academics actually gathered in a plush conference room and began their discussions, Kirmayer realized quickly that the GlaxoSmithKline representatives in attendance had no interest in touting their products to the group. Indeed there was little mention of the company's antidepressant drug Paxil, which was just a few months away from hitting the market in Japan. Instead they seemed much more interested in hearing from the assembled group. They were there to learn. "The focus was not on medications," Kirmayer remembers. "They were not trying to sell their drugs to us. They were interested in what we knew about how cultures shape the illness experience."

As Kirmayer got to know them during the conference, he realized that the drug company representatives weren't from the ranks of the advertising or marketing departments or the peppy salespeople. As best he could tell, these were highly paid private scholars who could hold their own in the most sophisticated discussion of postcolonial theory or the impact of globalization on the human mind. "These guys all had PhDs and were versed in the literature," Kirmayer said. "They were clearly soaking up what we had to say to each other on these topics."

The intense interest the GlaxoSmithKline brain trust showed in the topic of how culture shapes the illness experience made sense given the timing of the meeting. The class of antidepressant drugs known as selective serotonin reuptake inhibitors (SSRIs) had become the wonder drug of the 1990s, at least in terms of the profits they'd garnered for the drug companies. That year alone, in the leading regions for SSRIs, sales grew by 18 percent and totaled over thirteen billion dollars. Most of those sales were still in the United States, but there was wide agreement that lucrative international markets had yet to be tapped.

Indeed it was somewhat remarkable that none of the best-selling SSRIs had been launched in Japan. This was more than twelve years after Prozac became available for prescription in the United States. What caused this uncharacteristic timidity on the part of these pharmaceutical giants? It certainly wasn't that the Japanese eschewed Western drugs. To the contrary, U.S.-based companies at the time were exporting upwards of fifty billion dollars in medications to the country each year. It was said that Japanese patients felt underserved if they didn't come away from a doctor's visit with at least a couple of prescriptions.

But Eli Lilly, then the out-front world leader in the SSRI horse race with Prozac, had decided in the early 1990s not to pursue the Japanese market because executives in the company believed that the Japanese people wouldn't accept the drug. More precisely, they wouldn't want to accept the disease. "The people's attitude toward depression was very negative," explained a spokeswoman for Eli Lilly to the *Wall Street Journal.* She was referring to the fact that the Japanese had a fundamentally different conception of depression than in the West, one that made it unlikely that a significant number of people in Japan would want to take a drug associated with the disease.

Most other SSRI manufacturers followed Eli Lilly's lead and held off as well. Getting drugs approved in Japan was a costly gamble. The rules at the time required that drugs already on the market in Western countries had to be retested in large-scale human trials using an exclusively Japanese population. That meant years of effort and millions of dollars spent, with the distinct possibility that the drug might fail the trial. No company wanted to make such an investment if no market existed for the drug.

The Japanese pharmaceutical company Meiji Seika was the first to break from the pack, working through the decade to run Japanese trials on the SSRI Luvox, which it had licensed from the Swedish company Solvay. After reading Peter Kramer's 1993 book *Listening to Prozac,* Meiji's president, Ichiro Kitasato, sensed an unexplored opportunity in the Japanese marketplace. "People in the company said there are too few patients in Japan," he told a reporter in 1996. "But I looked at the U.S. and Europe and thought this is sure to be a big market."

GlaxoSmithKline was the next to get in the race. In the years prior to the 2000 conference in Kyoto, the company had spent an immense amount of money and resources jumping through the regulatory and bureaucratic hoops to get the green light to put Paxil on the market in the country. Having watched Prozac dominate the American market in the late 1980s, drug company executives knew the advantages of early market share, and GlaxoSmithKline didn't want Luvox to be the only SSRI in Japan.

But both companies faced the same problem: there was no guarantee that Japanese doctors would prescribe the drug or that the population would be interested in taking it. The problem was that the profession of psychiatry in Japan, unlike in the West, seldom ministered to the walking worried; rather they focused almost exclusively on the severely mentally ill. Consequently, talk therapy was all but nonexistent in the country. For the small percentage of the population diagnosed with a debilitating mental illness, long hospital stays were the norm. The average stay in a mental hospital in Japan was over a year, versus just ten days in the United States. So although there was a psychiatric term for depression in Japan, *utsubyô,* what it described was a mental illness that was as chronic and devastating as schizophrenia. *Utsubyô* was the sort of illness that would make it impossible to hold down a job or have a semblance of a normal life. Worse yet, at least for the sales prospects of Paxil in Japan, *utsubyô* was considered a rare disorder.

At the Kyoto meeting Kirmayer began to understand the company's intense interest in the question of how cultures shape the illness experience. To make Paxil a hit in Japan, it would not be enough to corner the small market of those diagnosed with *utsubyô.* The objective was to influence, at the most fundamental level, the Japanese understanding of sadness and depression. In short, they were learning how to market a disease.

To have the best chance of shifting the Japanese public's perception about the meaning of depression, GlaxoSmithKline needed a deep and sophisticated understanding of how those beliefs had taken shape. This was why, Kirmayer came to realize, the company had invited him and his colleagues and treated them like royalty. GlaxoSmithKline needed help solving a cultural puzzle that might be worth billions of dollars.

Judging from the records of the conference, it's clear that the company got its money's worth. During the meetings eminent scholars and researchers gave insightful presentations on subjects ranging from the history of psychiatry in Japan to the Japanese public's changing attitudes about mental illness. The prominent Japanese psychiatrists in attendance were particularly helpful in framing the state of the public's current beliefs about depression and anxiety disorders.

Osamu Tajima, a professor at the Department of Mental Health at Kyorin University and a leading Tokyo psychiatrist, told the assembled group of a rising public concern about the high suicide rates in Japan. He described how dozens of middle-aged men each year hike deep into the so-called suicide forests in the foothills of

Mt. Fuji with lengths of rope to hang themselves. He described how service along the Central Line Railway in Tokyo was routinely disrupted by office workers leaping in front of commuter trains.

Tajima also gave a detailed description of how psychiatric services were structured within the overall health care apparatus of Japan. Services were in the midst of a critical change, he reported. There was a burgeoning concern in the population about mood disorders and the need for social attention to suicide rates and depression. He also documented how the Western definition and symptom checklist for depression—thanks to the influence of the *DSM* in the profession—was steadily gaining ground among younger psychiatrists and doctors in Japan. "Japanese psychiatry is undergoing a period of important change," he concluded, which was certainly good news for GlaxoSmithKline. He was upbeat about the changes heralded by the standardization of psychiatry around the world. "Adoption of internationally standardized diagnostic criteria and terminology in psychiatry will provide additional advances in assessing prevalence and facilitating accurate diagnosis." He was also clearly impressed with the scientific advances in drug treatments that were soon to come to his country. "New and effective treatment options," he said, "most notably the SSRIs, will contribute to reducing the burden of depression and anxiety disorders in Japanese society."

After lunch on the second day of the conference, it was Kirmayer's turn to speak. He had written many papers in his career documenting the differing expressions of depression around the world and the meaning hidden in those differences. He had found that every culture has a type of experience that is in some ways parallel to the Western conception of depression: a mental state and set of behaviors that relate to a loss of connectedness to others or a decline in social status or personal motivation. But he had also found that cultures have unique expressions, descriptions, and understandings for these states of being.

He told the assembled scholars and drug company representatives of how a Nigerian man might experience a culturally distinct form of depression by describing a peppery feeling in his head. A rural Chinese farmer might speak only of shoulder or stomachaches. A man in India might talk of semen loss or a sinking heart or feeling hot. A Korean might tell you of "fire illness," which is experienced as a burning in the gut. Someone from Iran might talk of tightness in the chest, and an American Indian might describe the experience of depression as something akin to loneliness.

Kirmayer had observed that cultures often differ in what he called "explanatory models" for depression-like states. These cultural beliefs and stories have the effect of directing the attention of individuals to certain feelings and symptoms and away from others. In one culture someone feeling an inchoate distress might be prompted to search for feelings of unease in his gut or in muscle pain; in another place or time, a different type of symptom would be accepted as legitimate. This interplay between the expectations of the culture and the experience of the individual leads to a cycle of symptom amplification. In short, beliefs about the cause, symptomatology, and course of an illness such as depression tended to be self-fulfilling. Explanatory models created the culturally expected experience of the disease in the mind of the sufferer. Such differences, Kirmayer warned the group, tended to be overlooked when clinicians or researchers employed the symptom checklists relating to the *DSM* diagnosis of depression.

Understanding these differences is critical, however, because culturally distinct symptoms often hold precious clues about the causes of the distress. The American Indian symptom of feeling lonely, for instance, likely reflects a sense of social marginalization. A Korean who feels the epigastric pain of fire illness is expressing distress over an interpersonal conflict or a collective experience of injustice.

The wide variety of symptoms wasn't the only difference. Critically, not everyone in the world agreed that thinking of such experiences as an illness made sense. Kirmayer documented how feelings and symptoms that an American doctor might categorize as depression are often viewed in other cultures as something of a "moral compass," prompting both the individual and the group to search for the source of the social, spiritual, or moral discord. By applying a one-size-fits-all notion of depression around the world, Kirmayer argued, we run the risk of obscuring the social meaning and response the experience might be indicating.

Indeed, around the world, it is the Western conception of depression, in particular the American version of the disease, that is the most culturally distinctive. Kirmayer told the group that Americans are unique both in being willing to openly express distressful emotions and feelings to strangers and in our penchant for viewing psychological suffering as a health care issue. Because people in other cultures find social and moral meaning in such internal distress, they often seek relief exclusively from family members or community elders or local spiritual leaders. The idea of seeking help from a doctor or mental health professional outside one's social circle has traditionally made little sense.

The drug company representatives listened closely to Kirmayer's presentation and thanked him heartily afterward. To this day, he's not entirely sure what they took away from his presentation. In the end Kirmayer's comments could have been taken in two ways. On the one hand, they could be seen as a warning to respect and protect the cultural diversity of human suffering. In this way, he was like a botanist presenting a lecture to a lumber company on the complex ecology of the forest. On the other hand, he might have told the GlaxoSmithKline representatives exactly what they wanted to hear:

that cultural conceptions surrounding illnesses such as depression could be influenced and shifted over time. He made that point clearly in the conclusion of the paper he wrote based on his presentation:

> The clinical presentation of depression and anxiety is a function not only of patients' ethnocultural backgrounds, but of the structure of the health care system they find themselves in and the diagnostic categories and concepts they encounter in mass media and in dialogue with family, friends and clinicians.

In the globalizing world, he reported, these conceptions are

> in constant transaction and transformation across boundaries of race, culture, class, and nation. In this context, it is important to recognize that psychiatry itself is part of an international subculture that imposes certain categories on the world that may not fit equally well everywhere and that never completely captures the illness experience and concerns of patients.

In other words, cultural beliefs about depression and the self are malleable and responsive to messages that can be exported from one culture to another. One culture can reshape how a population in another culture categorizes a given set of symptoms, replace their explanatory model, and redraw the line demarcating normal behaviors and internal states from those considered pathological.

Kirmayer's appreciation of the irony of his brief encounter with GlaxoSmithKline has only grown over the years since he gave that presentation. "People like me got into cultural psychiatry because we were interested in differences between cultures—even treasured those differences in the same way a biologist treasures ecological diversity," Kirmayer told me. "So it's certainly ironic that cultural psychiatrists sometimes end up being handmaidens to these global marketing machines that are intent on manipulating cultural differences . . . in order to capitalize on those changes."

I asked Kirmayer how clear it was to him that GlaxoSmithKline was interested in changing notions of depression in Japan. "It was very explicit. What I was witnessing was a multinational pharmaceutical corporation working hard to redefine narratives about mental health," he said. "These changes have far-reaching effects, informing the cultural conceptions of personhood and how people conduct their everyday lives. And this is happening on a global scale. These companies are upending long-held cultural beliefs about the meaning of illness and healing."

The consensus paper produced to summarize the Kyoto conference provided both an action plan and a marketing piece for GlaxoSmithKline. In that paper the International Consensus Group on Depression and Anxiety warned that depression was vastly underestimated in Japan but that Western scientific advances would soon be on hand to help. "Clinical evidence supports the use of SSRIs as first-line therapy for depression and anxiety disorders," the paper concludes.

Looking back, Kirmayer can now see how the company used the conference as the beginning of its broader marketing strategy; its representatives identified the cultural challenges and fleshed out the resonant cultural notes the company would attempt to play in the critical coming months and years. Among those themes were that suicide in Japan was an indicator of undertreated depression; that Western SSRIs represented proven scientific advances in treatment; that primary care physicians should use simple three-minute surveys to help diagnose mental illness; that patients not meeting the criteria for depression should still be considered sick; and that the Japanese should be helped to reconceive social stress related to work and industrialization as signs of depression that should be treated with SSRIs. These confident conclusions would prove the foundation on which GlaxoSmithKline would begin to change the culture of Japan.

Psychiatry in the Time of Cholera

The rapid rise of the depression narrative in Japan, which took place over the next few years, is remarkable in many respects. The marketing campaign of GlaxoSmithKline and other SSRI makers set off a seismic shift in the culture, the aftershocks of which are still being felt. And just as earthquakes are the expression of tectonic pressures that build slowly over decades, there were unseen forces in the cultural history of Japan that laid the groundwork for Glaxo-SmithKline's remarkable success.

To understand how GlaxoSmithKline was so successful in selling depression in Japan at the beginning of this millennium, it's important to spend some time with a guide who knows the historical lay of the land. Ironically the person who best understands the cultural history of depression in Japan turns out to be none other than Junko Kitanaka, the grad student who was barred from the conference in 2000. In the years since, she finished her award-winning dissertation, "Society in Distress: The Psychiatric Production of Depression in Contemporary Japan," and has taken up an associate professorship at Keio University, an institution often compared with American Ivy League schools.

A visitor to the university will quickly notice that Keio's architects were intent on giving the place an Oxford–Ivy League flavor. At the Mita campus where Kitanaka works, campus gates are set in arches in red brick buildings and paths run into open courtyards filled with huge ginkgo trees that turn a luminescent yellow in the fall. As the style of the architecture suggests, Western influence on Japanese academia, particularly science and medicine, is hardly new.

When I asked Kitanaka how far back in time it was necessary to go to begin tracking the Western influence on mental health trends in Japan, she suggested that a good starting point was toward the end of the nineteenth century. This was when ideas of German neuropsychiatry and notions of neurasthenia—the disease of frayed nerves—first began to filter into Japanese professional and popular culture.

Cultures are most susceptible to outside ideas about the nature of the human mind at times of social change and upheaval, and the second half of the nineteenth century was just such a time in Japan. The Edo era—the rule of the shogun warlords—was at an end. For the previous 250 years Japan had stayed relatively isolated from many cultural trends and forces in the West, including those in science and medicine. During the long Edo era the population of Japan had thought of health mostly in terms of *yojo*, a set of concepts imported from China sometime between the seventh and tenth centuries. *Yojo* connected health with diet, mental control, exercise, and sexual restraint. It focused less on the control of disease or longevity and more on issues of social health, including morality, culture, and education.

During this time the concept that most closely tracked modern notions of depression would have been *utsushô,* which described the stagnation of vital energy, or *qi.* This stagnation or blockage could come from a combination of emotions, social conflict, loss, or the changing physiology of the body. Critically, as Kitanaka points out, the meaning of *utsushô* went beyond the narrow category of a mental disease. As portrayed in plays and popular books of the time, *utsushô* described a complex interaction between social forces, emotions, and physiology. The person affected by *utsushô* was not considered sick and did not necessarily seek a cure for his symptoms; rather it was sometimes expected that those affected would have to look for the social or moral meaning in their distress.

As the rule of the shoguns was replaced with that of the emperor, Japan began to open up to ideas from Europe and the United States. The Japanese public's acceptance of psychiatry as a legitimate field of science and mental health largely paralleled the growing influence of Western medicine.

It was the cholera epidemics, which began in 1859 and plagued the nation for the rest of the century, that were critical in breaking the hold of the *yojo* beliefs regarding health. These deadly epidemics terrified the population. Thousands died. The sick and those thought to be infected were hauled away to hospitals under police guard. Whole neighborhoods were sealed off and quarantined. According to Kitanaka, the state used the outbreaks to justify the creation of an imposing network of local government controls that claimed authority from Western advances in medicine. Improvements in sanitary conditions and public hygiene did appear to limit the cholera epidemics, and the success was taken as proof that European and Western knowledge about health and illness had validity. Traditional beliefs surrounding *yojo* were increasingly replaced by newer ideas of *eisei*, which encouraged the population to think of health as something that must be actively and carefully cultivated by following scientifically approved hygienic practices.

In choosing which Western public health models to follow, health ministers in the Japanese government were particularly taken with the German model, which promoted the idea that the individual and the society were best thought of as a single organism, each dependent on the health of the other. As more and more Japanese doctors and public health officials studied advances in German medical practices, the burgeoning science of neuropsychiatry was bound to follow. It wasn't long before many of Japan's most promising psychiatrists were making pilgrimages to Germany to find mentors among the ranks of the famous neuropsychiatrists of the day.

Those German doctors were focusing their attention on the severely mentally ill, especially patients with psychotic symptoms related to schizophrenia or manic depression. For the most part they believed that such dramatic mental illnesses were caused by malfunctions somewhere in the brain or nervous system and were likely the result of inherited predispositions. Following these interests, the first psychiatrists in Japan also focused their ministrations on those with severe psychotic symptoms.

Kitanaka shows that, as the cholera epidemic introduced the Japanese public to Western notions of medicine, Western psychiatry was carried into public consciousness through crisis. That crisis was the combination of rapid social changes at the end of the nineteenth century that included urbanization, the Industrial Revolution, and three wars within thirty years. Government officials and social commentators expressed increasing concern during this time over rising social problems such as increased juvenile delinquency and the disappearance of traditional practices and values. The government produced reports on rising suicide rates and the discontent of the working class. And just as Western-oriented medical doctors consulted with government officials to control the outbreaks of cholera, psychiatrists gave advice on the social discontent of the time. Newly minted psychiatrists in Japan, trained in German neuropsychiatry, suddenly found that they had a voice in these public debates.

In popular lectures and newspaper and magazine articles, these psychiatrists began to introduce new ideas into the popular culture. The people learned about hysteria in women, mental hygiene, and antisocial personalities. Given the uneasiness about the new realities of industrialization and urban living, there was intense interest and debate on these topics. Kitanaka cites one prominent intellectual who wrote in the early part of the twentieth century that the new medical knowledge had brought to light many ailments that the people had never heard of and that had previously gone unnoticed. The people, he said, were now "constantly worried over the slightest changes in their health" and had consequently become "more vulnerable to illness."

Japan's First Mental Health Epidemic

Of the many ideas being imported from those Western advances in psychiatric thinking, one in particular struck a chord with the Japanese population. Riding on its recent popularity in the United States and Europe, neurasthenia was introduced to the Japanese public as an illness of modernity.

Writing in professional and popular forums, Japanese psychiatrists and others knowledgeable about Western illness categories carefully explained to the public that neurasthenia (translated as *shinkeisuijaku*) was a disease of the nerves. The idea that the body had nerve pathways, often described as tiny electrical cables, was a new one for the Japanese, but the notion quickly became conventional wisdom. The metaphor often employed to describe this new condition was that of electric streetcars. Just as a trolley would fail to function if its electric cables became worn or broken, so too could human wiring fray and malfunction from overuse.

What made neurasthenia different from other psychiatric illnesses studied by Japanese psychiatrists at the time was that it was not a disorder of the severely mentally ill but of the common man. "The rise of neurasthenia," Kitanaka says, "was the first instance of the broad-scale medicalization of everyday distress in Japan." She found remarkable parallels between the rise of neurasthenia at the beginning of the twentieth century and the introduction of the Western conception of depression at the beginning of the twenty-first.

Neurasthenia, she believes, became a compelling social narrative in Japan because it distilled and gave a name to the inchoate anxiety of the times. Commentators connected the disease with all manner of troubling trends, including increased marketplace competition, excessive studying, smoking, drug abuse, labor inequities, rising crime rates, and juvenile delinquency.

The excitement surrounding the diagnosis of neurasthenia came not only from the mental health professionals of the time but from popular culture as well. Articles, pamphlets, and books provided guides to self-diagnosis, symptom lists, and suggestions for which specific groups should be considered particularly vulnerable. People were told to be on the lookout for symptoms: insomnia, ringing in the ears, lack of concentration, stomach pains, eye fatigue, and the feeling that a heavy pot covered one's head. A brisk market in pills and potions to cure the illnesses soon sprang up.

Unlike other mental illnesses being discussed in popular culture at the time, this one carried little social stigma. Indeed, because neurasthenia was at first considered an illness of the elites, the diagnosis became somewhat trendy. An article in an intellectual magazine circa 1902 was headlined "Neurasthenia: Operators, Writers, Government Officials, and Students, Read This." The assumption was that those employed in positions requiring strenuous intellectual labor were dangerously taxing their nerves. "The media initially depicted it as an inevitable outcome for people on the forefront of the process of modernization, for whom exhausted nerves even became a mark of distinction," Kitanaka explains. "An unprecedented number of cases of neurasthenia among elites, including government officials, company executives, university professors and artists began to be reported."

The belief that neurasthenia was a disease of the elites and intellectuals no doubt helped with the wide acceptance of the illness in Japan. By the early years of the twentieth century, however, it was not only the elites on the front lines of cultural change who were claiming this disease of modernity. In 1902 an article reported that fully one-third of patients visiting hospitals for consultations were suffering from this new disease. Large and diverse segments of the population were also reporting or being diagnosed as having frayed nerves. Neurasthenia was suddenly being referred to as Japan's "national disease."

But although the Japanese people seemed willing to accept, even idolize, this disease when it was only in an elite population, they were less sanguine when large numbers of regular citizens also invoked the diagnosis. With tens of thousands claiming the illness, the country was poised for a backlash.

Kitanaka identified one early sign of change in the debate surrounding a single suicide that caught the public's attention. In 1903 a young student named Misao Fujimura carved a poem in a tree near Nikko, a popular scenic area north of Tokyo. The message in the brief verse was that life was "incomprehensible." When he finished, he walked to a local waterfall renowned for its beauty and leaped to his death.

Those who wrote about his suicide in the years afterward fell into two broad categories. There were many artists and intellectuals who saw such suicides as having great social and philosophical meaning. Fueling the rise of the neurasthenia diagnosis was a popular idea that some Japanese were too pure of heart to live with the conflicts, compromises, and demands of modern life. Misao's suicide was a brave act, some prominent thinkers suggested, committed by a young man freeing himself from the mental torture of modernity. This understanding of his actions was in line with a long Japanese tradition of viewing suicide as an act of personal resolve. Just as neurasthenia was considered a mark of distinction among certain elite groups, suicides among similar groups were often excused or even admired as expressions of the purity of the Japanese character.

But as the diagnosis of neurasthenia began to rise exponentially, some prominent doctors and officials stepped forward to challenge the social status given individuals like poor Misao. Kitanaka cites a speech to psychiatrists reprinted in a 1906 issue of the *Journal of Neurology*, in which the statesman Shigenobu Okuma took a harder line:

> These days, young students talk about such stuff as the "philosophy of life" [applause from the floor]. They confront important and profound problems of life, are defeated, and develop neurasthenia. Those who jump off of a waterfall or throw themselves in front of a train are weak-minded. They do not have a strong mental constitution and develop mental illness, dying in the end. How useless they are! Such weak-minded people would only cause harm even if they remained alive [applause].

Prominent psychiatrists also began to question the diagnosis. In a book on mental illness published in 1912 a professor at Kyushu University wrote that those who suffered from neurasthenia were "born with an inherent weakness in the brain" and had only "half the mental capacity of a normal person." Not everyone who had a mentally taxing job, other psychiatrists pointed out, developed the disease; thus there must be something fundamentally wrong with the affected individuals to make them vulnerable.

Psychiatrists began to offer up new categories and formulations. They began to talk of the difference between the few who had "true neurasthenia" and a larger number of people who were burdened with a type of nervous disposition. This sort of disposition was not caused by the overwork and mental stress that came with high-profile elite jobs but came from an inherited abnormal personality that made the sufferer incapable of withstanding the everyday challenges of a normal life.

Looking back on the debate, it seems as if acceptance of neurasthenia had been so successful that psychiatrists felt obligated to *restigmatize* this mental disorder in hopes of limiting its adoption. By the end of World War II the diagnosis had almost completely gone out of style among both psychiatrists and the population at large. A new generation of psychiatrists wrote papers and gave presentations dismissing neurasthenia by suggesting that the thousands of patients who had claimed to suffer from the illness had either been misdiagnosed by uninformed doctors or were malingerers trying to get time off work.

The Culture of Sadness

During the early part of the twentieth century the concept of depression remained attached to the diagnosis of severe manic depression imported from those German neuropsychiatrists. It wasn't until after World War II that depression became a disease category of its own. There was nothing mild about this conception of depression. This so-called endogenous depression was a crippling type of psychosis believed to be caused by a genetic abnormality. Professors of psychiatry at the time often explained endogenous depression using the metaphor of an internal alarm clock. "According to this model, the depressed person is like someone carrying a psychotic time bomb, for whom depression begins when the internal clock goes off and ends after it runs its course," Kitanaka explains. Endogenous depression expressed itself only in individuals with that ticking alarm clock and wasn't connected to external causes.

At the same time Kitanaka shows that another idea was gaining ground in Japan's mental health community. The personality *typus melancholicus* was introduced in the early 1960s by a professor of clinical psychopathology from Heidelberg named Hubert Tellenbach. This idea never caught on in the United States and rather quickly became dated in Germany, but it influenced psychiatric thinking in Japan. As Tellenbach first described it, someone with a melancholic personality possessed a highly developed sense of orderliness as well as "exceptionally high demands regarding one's own achievements." *Typus melancholicus* mirrored a particularly respected personality style in Japan: those who were serious, diligent, and thoughtful and expressed great concern for the welfare of other individuals and the society as a whole. Such people, the theory went, were prone to feeling overwhelming sadness when cultural upheaval disordered their lives and threatened the welfare of others.

Neither endogenous depression nor the melancholic personality type were of great concern to the general public at the time. Because endogenous depression was thought of as a psychotic state, akin to schizophrenia in severity, it carried a severe stigma and was considered rare. As for the melancholic personality type, its association with such prized Japanese traits as orderliness and high achievement meant that having such a sadness-prone personality was something not to be feared but aspired to.

This absence of a category parallel with the modern Western-style depression persisted for many years. When the *DSM-III* was first translated into Japanese in 1982, the diagnosis of depression, with its two-week threshold for low mood, was widely criticized among Japanese psychiatrists as far too expansive and vague to be of any use. Prominent psychiatrists believed, in short, that the description did not amount to a meaningful mental illness.

Indeed, as Kirmayer has pointed out, in the late twentieth century no word in Japanese had the same connotations as the word "depression" in English. Consider the various words and phrases that have often been translated into English as "depression." *Utsubyô* describes a severe, rare, and debilitating condition that usually required inpatient care and thus was not much of a match for the common English word "depression." *Yuutsu*, which describes grief as well as a general gloominess of the body and spirit, was in common use. There was also *ki ga fusagu*, which refers to blockages in vital energy. Similarly, *ki ga meiru* is the leakage or loss of such energy. Although each of these words and phrases had overlaps with the English word "depression," there were also critical differences. The experiences these words describe do not exist only in the thoughts and emotions but encompass full-body sadness. As such, the Japanese person who felt *yuutsu* or *ki ga fusagu* was likely to describe it in terms of bodily sensations, such as having headaches or chest pains or feeling heavy in the head.

Not only did Japanese ideas of sadness include both the body and the mind but, metaphorically at least, they sometimes existed beyond the self. The experience of *yuutsu* in particular contained connotations of the physical world and the weather. A young Japanese researcher named Junko Tanaka-Matsumi, studying at the University of Hawaii in the mid-1970s, conducted a simple word-association test on a group of Japanese college students and compared the results to Caucasian American college students. The American students were asked to respond with three words that they connected with "depression." The Japanese students were asked to do the same with *yuutsu*.

The top ten word associations for the native Japanese were

1. Rain
2. Dark

3. Worries
4. Gray
5. Suicide
6. Solitude
7. Exams
8. Depressing
9. Disease
10. Tiredness

For the Caucasian Americans, the top ten word associations were

1. Sad or sadness
2. Lonely or loneliness
3. Down
4. Unhappy
5. Moody
6. Low
7. Gloom
8. Failure
9. Upset
10. Anxious

Comparing these answers, Tanaka-Matsumi saw a notable difference. In the responses given by the Japanese natives, only a few of the words (such as "worries" and "solitude") were related to internal emotional states. On the other hand, the majority of the word associations supplied by the American students related to internal moods. The Japanese, in short, were looking outward to describe *yuutsu*, and the Americans were looking inward to describe depression. Tanaka-Matsumi believed that these were not simply linguistic differences but cultural "variations in the subjective meanings and *experience* of depression."

The Japanese and Americans weren't just talking about depression and sadness differently, she believed; they were *feeling* these states differently as well. What she saw reflected in the language was a difference between how Japanese and Americans conceived of the nature of the self. The word associations suggested that Americans experience the self as isolated within the individual mind. The Japanese, on the other hand, conceive of a self that is less individuated and more interconnected and dependent on social and environmental contexts. Feelings that Americans associate with depression have, in Japan, been wrapped up in a variety of cultural narratives that altered their meaning and the subjective experience for the individual.

Even as the *DSM* diagnosis of depression became more widely employed around the world during the 1980s, the experience of deep sadness and distress in Japan retained the characteristics of the premodern conception of both *utsushô* and the mid-twentieth-century idealization *typus melancholicus,* the idea that overwhelming sadness was natural, quintessentially Japanese, and, in some ways, an enlightened state.

As Kirmayer has documented, this was a culture that often idealized and prized states of melancholy. Feelings of overwhelming sadness were often venerated in television shows, movies, and popular songs. Kirmayer noted that *yuutsu* and other states of melancholy and sadness have been thought of as *jibyo,* that is, personal hardships that build character. Feelings that we might pathologize as depressive were often thought of in Japan as a source of moral meaning and self-understanding. He and others have connected this reverence to the Buddhist belief that suffering is more enduring and more definitive of the human experience than transient happiness.

Other cross-cultural scholars have also noticed this Japanese affinity for states of sadness. Studying menopause in Japan,

McGill Social Studies of Medicine professor Margaret Lock wrote:

> Feeling sad and reacting sensitively to losses, particularly of loved ones, is an idea that has a singular appeal in Japanese. The theater, a range of literature and indigenous popular songs, traditional and modern, positively wallow in nostalgia, sensation of grief and loss, and a sense of the impermanence of things. People cry freely (by North American and northern European standards) about separation and lost loved ones, but at the same time they seem to draw strength from these experiences, to tighten their bonds with those who remain among the living, and to reaffirm group solidarity.

This cultural embrace of sadness, Lock believes, might have been motivated by society's discouragement of other emotional states.

> Unlike anger and irritability, which both disrupt harmony and threaten the social order, sadness, grief, and melancholy are accepted as an inevitable part of human life and even welcomed at times for their symbolic value, as a reminder of the ephemeral nature of this world. An association between melancholy and the weather reinforces sad feelings as natural and unavoidable and hence as states not induced solely through human exchange.

Given these cultural currents, it makes sense that the first popular psychopharmacological medications adopted in the 1960s and 1970s were sedatives, whereas amphetamines and early mood enhancers were viewed with suspicion. As Lock implies, culturally designated pathological states are often the flipside of states a culture values. Along with the sedating drugs, Japanese quickly adopted disease categories describing social anxiety or aggression but resisted viewing deep and extended periods of sadness as a mental illness.

When the first SSRIs came online in the West, consequently, Japanese considered them harsh medications that exaggerated types of personality valued in the United States. A leading Japanese psychopharmacologist described how classes of drugs matched or ran afoul of different cultural narratives: "The Japanese system is much more modest and co-operative—people work together more. Against this background, amphetamines are much more of a problem than are the benzodiazepines; we are much more sensitive to the changes, the exaggeration of behavior, produced by the amphetamines. Sedative agents are seen as much less of a problem in Japan. . . . There is something of a preference for an agent that will be sedative rather than arousing, like, perhaps, Prozac."

"One society's enhancement of personality can be another's pathology or provocation," remarks Kirmayer. "Something like this may occur with Prozac, where the extraversion, gregariousness and pushiness that typify the life of a salesman in the USA may be associated with inappropriately brash and insensitive social behavior in Japan."

Given all these cultural forces, it is not surprising that major drug companies at first saw no market for SSRIs in Japan at the beginning of the 1990s. The psychiatric category of depression was not a widespread public concern, and the capacity to experience great sadness was considered not a burden but a mark of strength and distinction. That belief, combined with a suspicion of drugs that heightened moods or extraverted personality traits, made the market for SSRIs unpromising. Those public perceptions, however, were soon to change.

In the Lost Decade a Young Man Joins an Ad Firm

In the spring of 1990, 24-year-old Oshima Ichiro joined the Dentsu advertising agency, the largest company of its kind in the world. When he first showed up at Dentsu, Oshima was healthy and athletic. His fellow employees described him as honest, happy, and committed. Like many unmarried men, he lived with his mother, father, and brother. He had a girlfriend but no immediate plans to get married; establishing his career would come first. At Dentsu he was assigned the daunting task of handling public relations for more than forty corporate clients.

Because Kitanaka believes that the odyssey of young Oshima began a new understanding of depression and suicide in Japan, she recounts the story in great detail in her dissertation. Most of the following facts and insights are drawn from that document. Owing to the significance of the case, it is worth pausing to note the timing of his hiring in relation to the trajectory of the economy of Japan.

It was on the last trading day of 1989, just three months before Oshima started his new job, that the Japanese Nikkei index hit an all-time high. That index had nearly quadrupled in value over the previous five years. At the end of those go-go days, choice apartments in the Ginza district of Tokyo were going for nearly $100,000 per square foot. The Japanese economy was the envy of the world. It was a time when it seemed that any business could secure a loan and everyone with the willingness to work hard could ride the wave of prosperity.

But when stock traders got back to their posts at the beginning of January 1990, something had shifted. In the next days and weeks stocks began to slide, and then free-fall. By the time Oshima started his job in April there was something approaching panic in the financial markets.

As was true of many new hires, the sudden economic downturn steeled Oshima's resolve to prove his worth. He showed right away that he was willing to roll up his sleeves and dig into his considerable workload. He often spent the first eight hours of his workday just trying to juggle meetings and field phone calls. Staying at work after hours was the only way he could write the press releases and proposals his clients required. Just a few months into his job, he was coming home past midnight on most nights. On some mornings, when his colleagues showed up for work, it was clear that the harddriving Oshima had been at his desk the entire night. He took no days off.

In November 1990 his mother and father began to worry about his health. Oshima's eyes looked unfocused and he sometimes fell asleep while sitting with them at the kitchen table. In his contract, Oshima was promised ten days of vacation each year, and his parents suggested that he schedule some days to rest. But he refused. He felt that any days off would only increase the burden he would face when he got back to work. Anyway, he told them, he didn't think his boss would allow him the time off. Not knowing what else to do, his mother made him nutritious breakfasts in the morning and drove him to the train station to ease the burden of his hourlong commute.

After months at this sprinter's pace, cracks began to show in his behavior. At work small setbacks and mistakes brought on waves of self-loathing. "I'm no good as a human being," coworkers sometimes heard him saying out loud to himself. "I'm of no use."

The New Year brought no relief from the economic bad news or from Oshima's burdens. From its high in 1989, the Nikkei had lost nearly half of its value. Home prices were plummeting just as precipitously. The normally hardworking life in corporate Japan became even more intense. The frustration of Dentsu executives at their declining profits rolled down the chain of command, putting ever more pressure on the rank and file. At one late-night drinking binge at the office, Oshima's boss poured beer into his own shoe and demanded that Oshima drink it down. When he momentarily refused the request, his boss beat him.

By the summer of that year Oshima's workload had only gotten worse. On top of his regular duties, he was put in charge of a four-day conference for a client to be held in August. If he got home at all that summer, his parents remember, it was often simply to clean himself up before getting back on the train to the office. On the night before the beginning of the conference he managed to get home at 6 a.m. He was back at work less than four hours later to drive his boss to the site of the conference.

As they drove, his boss couldn't help but notice that Oshima seemed troubled. He drifted and swerved erratically from lane to lane. He mumbled incoherently, something about being possessed by spirits.

After a grueling four days at the conference, Oshima finally made his way back home at 6 a.m. on August 26. He looked so drawn and haggard that he promised his brother that he would go to the hospital that day. He called the office at 9 a.m. to tell them that he was sick and would not be in that day. Less than an hour later, his family found him dead. He had hanged himself in the bathroom.

When Oshima's parents' lawsuit against Dentsu came to court a few years after his death, newspaper editors and television producers featured the story prominently. It was an easy pick, given that the story had a clear antecedent. In the boom years of the 1980s hardworking Japanese businessmen sometimes collapsed and died at their desks after putting in weeks or months of overtime. In the press this was called *karoshi,* death from overwork, and reports on the trend had become popular. In the early 1990s suicides topped thirty thousand a year. This was between three and four times the number of Japanese killed in car accidents. The suicide trend became a concern to the general public and there was much debate over who or what was responsible. When Oshima's suicide came to light, journalists and editors immediately saw the story's potential. Headlines announced the new trend: *karojisatsu,* suicide from overwork. Because the Oshima family's lawsuit sought to assign blame for his death, it was tailor-made to become the focus of this public debate.

The lawyers for Oshima's parents argued that the stress of his job and his long hours brought on a depression that caused his death. As Kitanaka demonstrates, this form of depression was different from the endogenous depression in the Japanese psychiatric literature because it hadn't resulted from an inherited defect in Oshima's brain; rather it was brought on by the circumstances of his life. This was a type of depression that could strike anyone.

The newspapers followed each revelation of the case. There was, for instance, the mystery of just how many overtime hours young Oshima worked during his time at Dentsu. According to the time sheets he submitted to the company, his overtime ranged between twelve and twenty hours each week. Lawyers for the company pointed out that that level of commitment was hardly unusual in hardworking Japan, and it was certainly not the sort of workload that you'd expect would drive a healthy and ambitious young man to hang himself in the bathroom. To prove that he had worked much longer than he claimed, the lawyers for his parents relied on the records of the office night guards, who were required to make frequent checks of each floor of the building, noting the names of the employees at their desks. Based on that evidence, it was clear that Oshima was clocking a much more problematic *average* of forty-seven overtime hours per week.

Oshima's parents won their case. As the Dentsu lawyers appealed the verdict through the courts they continued to argue that the company should not be held liable because Oshima's depression was a result of a preexisting mental weakness. They were, in effect, arguing for a pre–*DSM-III* version of endogenous depression: Oshima wouldn't have become sick had he not had that alarm clock ticking inside his brain.

The different rulings of the higher courts, Kitanaka suggests, rather neatly reflect a culture in the process of changing its collective mind. The Tokyo High Court first reduced the amount of the compensation, concluding that Oshima's inborn mental stamina was at least part of the cause in his death. "Not everyone becomes depressed from being overworked or being in a stressful situation," the verdict read. "It cannot be denied that his . . . premorbid personality resulted in increasing the amount of his own work." Here the court held onto earlier notions prominent in Japanese psychiatry: that inborn pathological characteristics were the psychiatric equivalent of fate. The Supreme Court, however, rejected that lower court's ruling and argued that individual character—as long as it is within a normal spectrum—should not be considered in such a case. The ruling suggested that anyone, put under enough stress, could succumb to depression.

Thanks partly to the debate over Oshima's suicide, Kitanaka argues, the shift in public opinion during this period couldn't have been more dramatic. "When people first heard about the litigation, they would ask if it was the company, not the family, that was suing for the damage caused by the employee's suicide." Kitanaka cites one of the attorneys in the case, commenting, "When Japanese heard in the media of the plaintiff's victory, many came to hear, probably for the first time, that suicide could be caused by a mental illness called depression."

That Oshima's lawsuit might be the first time many Japanese connected suicide with depression is hard for a Westerner to comprehend. Most Americans would certainly assume that suicidal acts are nearly always caused by mental illness, most commonly depression. Indeed the Western SSRI manufacturers who were eyeing the Japanese market in the 1990s routinely invoked the high suicide rate as proof positive of an epidemic of depression in Japan.

Yet the Japanese public remained split as to whether suicide was an intentional act with moral or philosophical meaning or a desperate act of a mentally ill person. In many ways the public debate regarding why Oshima hanged himself picked up the public dialogue that took place almost a hundred years before, when Misao Fujimura jumped off the waterfall. Although many Japanese agreed that the high rate of suicide was a legitimate public health concern, there was not yet a consensus that the epidemic, or the act of suicide itself, was the result of mental illness. In Japanese history, literature, and movies there were many stories of the noble suicide, such as when Samurai warriors committed *seppuku* and World War II soldiers killed themselves to avoid capture. Psychiatrist Masao Miyamoto was not alone when he remarked in 1998 that he didn't see much of a connection between the rise of suicide and depression. Most of the reasons Japanese people kill themselves have nothing to do with depression, he argued. "A peculiarity of the Japanese is that they often die for the sake of the group," he said. "They die for shame." Wataru Tsurumi's *Complete Manual of Suicide*, published in 1993, was the modern embodiment of the Japanese public's intense interest in suicide. The book, written in flat, unemotional tones, is a guide to the ten most popular methods of suicide, including hanging, drowning, electrocution, and jumping from heights. The author awards a number of skulls to rate each method in categories such as painfulness, how much a nuisance you'll cause others, how much effort is required, and the likelihood of success.* The remark-

---

*The instructions are given in great detail. For potential jumpers, for example, the book recommends the Takashimadaira housing project and provides a map to help the reader find the place. The chapter on throwing oneself in front of a train recommends precisely where to stand on the platform and which express trains will do the quickest work. To combat these instructions, the transit authority has placed mirrors at strategic spots, following the theory that seeing one's reflection may dissuade one from jumping.

able sales of the book speak to a uniquely Japanese fascination. During the 1990s the book sold more than 1.2 million copies. If we can believe the author, the book was written not for shock value but from a deeply philosophical belief that suicide is a legitimate—and perfectly sane—act of personal will.

The story of young Oshima and several other prominent suicides from overwork put faces and personal stories on the growing public concern that Japan had ignored the mental health consequences of overwork. As was true at the turn of the nineteenth century, the end of the twentieth century was a disconcerting time for the people of Japan. Shameful bankruptcies were common and divorce and unemployment were on the rise. Just as at the end of the Edo era a hundred years before, the public was on the hunt to explain the distress being felt during these uncertain times.

The Japanese public's impression that the country was behind the times in addressing mental health got a boost after the devastating earthquake in the city of Kobe in January 1995.* The government response to the disaster was criticized by Western mental health experts for being lackluster on many fronts. Researchers from the United States were soon on the scene and garnered much press attention by suggesting that the population needed not just food and shelter but more attention paid to their emotional and mental health.

Several prominent Japanese psychiatrists and mental health advocates used the authority of the visiting mental health experts to make a broad argument that Japanese culture discouraged talking about emotionally loaded issues. "The comparison, quite unfavorable to Japan, was often made to the United States, where the emphasis on psychological issues is generally believed to be cultur-

---

*As discussed in chapter 2 this disaster also played a key role in the international spread of the PTSD diagnosis.

ally strong and given proper priority," the anthropologist Joshua Breslau reported. "One well-known newspaper critic noted that his friend told him how nearly everyone in U.S. cities has a psychological counselor."

A critical turning point came just three months after the Kobe quake. A TV producer named Kenichiro Takiguchi was browsing through the English-language section of a Tokyo bookstore and started to flip through a paperback copy of Peter Kramer's American best seller *Listening to Prozac*. Always on the lookout for good ideas for programs, he took the book to his bosses at Japan's largest television network and persuaded them to let him produce a fifty-minute special. The message of the special was similar to the beliefs made popular after the Kobe earthquake, namely, that Americans were far advanced in their recognition and treatment of emotional disorders such as depression and anxiety. The show hit a nerve. Millions watched and more than two thousand viewers called in afterward to praise the network for running the program.

Japanese psychiatrists were largely taken by surprise at this turn in public interest. Up to that point the public had eschewed the intrusion of psychiatry into daily life. As the small population of psychiatrists had mostly limited their practice to the severely mentally ill, the call to address common unhappiness and anxiety that came with bad economic times caught them off-guard. Like many people in the country up to that point, they had not considered unhappiness (or divorce or suicide) a mental health issue. They were in need of a new and compelling explanation for what was going on. Fortunately for them, GlaxoSmithKline and several other major psychopharmaceutical companies were just then preparing to throw them a lifeline.

Junk Science and First World Medicine

Kalman Applbaum, a professor at the University of Wisconsin in Milwaukee, is an anthropologist, but he doesn't study little-known tribes in far-off lands. His interest is closer at hand: the rituals and practices of international corporations. His specialty, the anthropology of the boardroom, has led to teaching posts both in anthropology departments and at business schools, including Harvard and Kellogg. He is also fluent in Japanese and often consults with companies interested in the Asian markets. When he heard in the late 1990s that major players in the pharmaceutical industry were attempting to introduce SSRIs to Japan, he knew he had the topic for his next set of research papers.

At the beginning of the new millennium, Applbaum went out of his way to visit the headquarters of GlaxoSmithKline, Lilly, and Pfizer, the major international players who were at various stages of trying to get their drugs into Japan. At the time both Pfizer and Lilly were playing catch-up to GlaxoSmithKline, which was just then launching Paxil in the country. Although he had to sign non-disclosure agreements promising that he wouldn't identify the executives by name or company affiliation, Applbaum managed to get remarkable access to the inner workings of these companies. Several of his former MBA students who were then working in these firms helped make key introductions, but in the end these executives proved more than willing to talk. When I asked Applbaum why they were so forthcoming, he told me it was simple: because of his business school credentials and his extensive experience in the Japanese market, they thought he might be able to give them some free advice.

Applbaum discovered that the companies intent on entering the SSRI market in Japan were not battling each other like Coke and

Pepsi for market share—or at least not at the beginning. Instead he found wide acknowledgment within the ranks of drug company executives that the best way for companies to create a market was for competing companies to join forces.

A critical player in this joint effort was the trade organization Pharmaceutical Manufacturers of America, or PhRMA, which functions as the national and international lobby and public relations organization for a coalition of major drug companies. In the late 1990s Applbaum found PhRMA working on a number of levels in Japan to influence what they considered to be a backward and bureaucratic drug approval process. As one PhRMA executive based in Chiyoda-Ku, Tokyo, told Applbaum, their job was to create "a market based upon competitive, customer choice and a transparent pricing structure that supports innovation." The lobby wanted drugs such as Paxil to be able to enter new markets based on "global, objective, scientific standards."

The more Applbaum talked to drug company insiders, the more righteous frustration he found. When he visited the offices of a leading SSRI manufacturer in November 2001, he discovered a wellspring of anger directed at what they perceived as Japanese resistance to pharmaceutical progress. These executives criticized scientific standards for clinical testing in Japan as "quite poor" and asserted that there was no "good clinical practice" in the country. Why, they asked Applbaum rhetorically, should their company be forced to retest these drugs in exclusively Japanese populations? The assumption was that the science behind the American human trials was unassailable—certainly better than anything the Japanese would attempt.

No doubt that annoyance at having to retest drugs was so intense because a couple of recent large-scale human trials of SSRIs in Japan had *failed* to show any positive effects. Drugs such as Pfizer's Zoloft, which were widely prescribed in the United States, had at least one large-scale human trial failure in Japan in the 1990s. Instead of considering the meaning of such results, the drug company executives railed at Japanese testing practices, calling them second rate. "There is no sense of urgency about patient need in Japan," one executive complained to Applbaum.

The Mega-Marketing of Depression

Although drug company executives clearly would have preferred to avoid the expensive and time-consuming process of retesting their SSRIs in Japan, they ultimately found a way to put those trials to good use as the first step in their marketing campaign. The drug makers often bought full-page ads in newspapers in the guise of recruiting test subjects. Applbaum believes that this was one of several savvy methods the drug companies employed to sidestep the prohibitions in Japan on marketing prescription drugs directly to the consumer. These advertisements, supposedly designed only to recruit people for the trials, were well worth the cost, as they both featured the brand name of the drug and promoted the idea of depression as a common ailment. One company scored even more public attention when it recruited a well-known actress to take part in the trials.

But getting the drug approved for market was only the first step. Talking with these executives, it became clear to Applbaum that they were intent on implementing a complex and multifaceted plan to, as he put it, "alter the total environment in which these drugs are or may be used." Applbaum took to calling this a "mega-marketing" campaign—an effort to shape the very consciousness of the Japanese consumer.

The major problem GlaxoSmithKline faced was that Japanese

psychiatrists and mental health professionals still translated the diagnosis of "depression" as *utsubyô*, and in the mind of many Japanese that word retained its association with an incurable and inborn depression of psychotic proportions. In hopes of softening the connotations of the word, the marketers hit upon a metaphor that proved remarkably effective. Depression, they repeated in advertising and promotional material, was *kokoro no kaze*, like "a cold of the soul." It is not clear who first came up with the phrase. It is possible that it originated from Kenichiro Takiguchi's prime-time special on depression. In that show, it was said that Americans took antidepressants the way other cultures took cold medicine.

Whatever its origin, the line *kokoro no kaze* appealed to the drug marketers, as it effectively shouldered three messages at the same time. First, it implied that *utsubyô* was not the severe condition it was once thought to be and therefore should carry no social stigma. Who would think less of someone for having a cold? Second, it suggested that the choice of taking a medication for depression should be as simple and worry-free as buying a cough syrup or an antihistamine. Third, the phrase communicated that, like common colds, depression was ubiquitous. Everyone, after all, from time to time suffers from a cold.

Although advertising couldn't mention particular drugs, companies could run spots in the guise of public service announcements encouraging people to seek professional help for depression. In these ads SSRI makers attempted to distance depression further from the endogenous depression as it was understood by Japanese psychiatrists for most of the century. One GlaxoSmithKline television advertisement showed an attractive young woman standing in a green field, asking, "How long has it been? How long has it been since you began to worry that it might be depression?" The scene then shows a woman on an escalator and then a middle-aged office worker staring out a bus window. The voiceover then recommends that if you've been feeling down for a month, "do not endure it. Go see a doctor."

The subtext of the ad is clear to Kitanaka. It presents depression as "intentionally ambiguous and ill-defined, applicable to the widest possible population and to the widest possible range of discomforts. . . . The only feature that distinguishes depression as a 'disease' from an ordinary depressed mood seems to be the length of time (one month) that the person has experienced these 'symptoms.'"

Depression was so broadly defined by the marketers that it clearly encompassed classic emotions and behaviors formerly attributed to the melancholic personality type. The label of depression then took on some laudable characteristics, such as being highly sensitive to the welfare of others and to discord within the family or group. Being depressed in this way became a testament to one's deeply empathic nature.

To get these messages out to the Japanese public, the SSRI makers employed a variety of techniques and avenues. Company marketers quickly reproduced and widely disseminated articles in newspapers and magazines mentioning the rise of depression, particularly if those pieces touted the benefits of SSRIs. The companies also sponsored the translation of several best-selling books first published in the United States on depression and the use of antidepressants.

Given all the ways that GlaxoSmithKline and the other SSRI makers managed to make the average Japanese aware of their drugs, the official ban on direct-to-consumer marketing became almost meaningless. If there was any doubt about this, one only had to look at how these companies used the Internet. "The best way to reach patients today is not via advertising but the Web," one Tokyo-based marketing manager told Applbaum. "The Web basically circumvents [direct-to-consumer advertising] rules, so there is no need to be concerned over these. People go to the company website and take a quiz to see whether they might have depression. If yes, then they go to the doctor and ask for medication."

The mega-marketing campaign often came in disguised forms, such as patient advocacy groups that were actually created by the drug companies themselves. The website utu-net.com, which appeared to be a coalition of depressed patients and their advocates, was funded by GlaxoSmithKline, although visitors to the site would have had no clue of the connection. What they would have found was a series of articles on depression driving home the key points of the campaign, including the idea that it was a common illness and that antidepressants bring the brain's natural chemistry back into balance.

The public interest in the new diagnosis brought a remarkable amount of media attention. Often in back-to-back months, the major magazines *Toyo Keizai* and *DaCapo* ran pieces on depression and the new drugs. In 2002 a leading Japanese business magazine ran a twenty-six-page cover story encouraging businesspeople to seek professional help for depression. The article rather perfectly mirrored the key points of the SSRI makers' mega-marketing campaign and in many ways reflected the early conceptions of neurasthenia a century before. The article suggested that it was the more talented and hard-charging workers who were the most susceptible to depression. Estimates of how many Japanese secretly suffered from depression, which ranged from 3 to 17 percent of the population, seemed to increase every month.

The distress caused by the long-ailing economy also proved to be a useful selling point. GlaxoSmithKline promoted the idea that there was an enormous economic cost for untreated depression, which could be counted in lost man-hours and decreased productivity. In this way, the lure of the drug, especially to the younger generation, was tied to ideas about competition in the global marketplace. One Japanese psychiatrist was quoted in a local newspaper describing SSRIs as "drugs that can transform minus thinking into plus thinking" and that "can help a person live tough," like financially successful Americans.

The SSRI makers made much of one public relations windfall in particular. It was rumored for years (and finally confirmed by the Imperial Household Agency) that Crown Princess Masako suffered from depression. Soon it was revealed that she was taking antidepressants as part of her treatment. This was a huge boost for the profile of depression and SSRIs in the country. Princess Masako's personal psychiatrist was none other than Yutaka Ono, one of the field's leaders that GlaxoSmithKline had feted at the Kyoto conference in 2001.

As a marketing line, there was one problem with the phrase *kokoro no kaze:* the metaphor lacked a sense of urgency about the condition. After all, one rarely rushes to the doctor with a cold. Worse yet, medicating a cold was always optional, as the illness goes away rather quickly on its own.

To counter this aspect of the metaphor, the drug companies leveraged the population's growing concern over the high suicide rates. The medical anthropologist Emiko Namihira reported that SSRI makers were funding studies to prove the link between depression and suicide. Those studies that showed a connection were reprinted in pamphlet form and reported to national media outlets as breaking news. Studies that failed to show a connection could simply be ignored. The founder of the Mood Disorders Association of Japan claimed in the *Japan Times* that "90 percent of those who commit suicide are considered to suffer from one kind of mental illness or another, and 70 percent of suicides are attributable to depression." Without medical attention, the message went, this "cold of the soul" could kill you.

When taken together, the messages advanced by GlaxoSmith-

Kline during their rollout of Paxil don't always make sense. Previous notions of endogenous depression were employed only sparingly in order to evoke the seriousness of the disorder. On the other hand, they were happy to associate this new conception of depression with the Japanese veneration of the melancholic personality, even though that didn't particularly jibe with the parallel message that this was an illness caused by an imbalance of serotonin. Neither did the message that overwork could spark depression mesh with the idea that individuals should counter such social distress by taking a medication that changed their brain chemistry. If it was unrealistic social demands that were the cause of distress in the population, why should the individual be taking the pills? In the end, however, the coherence of these various messages took second place to their effectiveness.

Speeding the Evolution

After the Kobe earthquake in Japan there was growing consensus in the country that the West, and the United States in particular, had a deeper scientific understanding of pathological emotional states such as PTSD and depression. Responding to this insecurity, the advertisements, websites, waiting room brochures, and other materials produced by the drug companies played up the idea that SSRIs represented the cutting edge of medical science. These drugs, which were said to rebalance the natural chemicals in the brain, would bring Japan up to date.

GlaxoSmithKline worked very hard to win over the most prominent medical researchers and psychiatrists in the country and keep them on message. Their inclusion at lavish conferences such as the one Kirmayer attended was just a taste of the incentives offered. Drug companies offered grants to sponsor research on their drugs; those researchers who produced results favorable to the drugs found themselves with new offers of research funding. Research that showed the drug in question to be both safe and effective was trumpeted by the company and the researchers often paid as consultants. In addition, researchers were given honoraria for speaking about their findings at drug company–sponsored professional conferences. Influence over the prominent scientists and researchers in Japan was so pervasive that Applbaum concluded that these scientists and doctors had been basically "commandeered into a kind of market research by pharmaceutical companies. The research simultaneously serves as publicity for the essentially predetermined consumer need."

It is important to note that the drug company executives whom Applbaum interviewed didn't present themselves as people driven only by profits. Rather these men and women saw themselves as acting with the best of intentions, motivated by the belief that their drugs represented the proud march of scientific progress across the world. They styled themselves as people fighting depression, anxiety, and social phobia—diseases that remained cruelly untreated in Japan and elsewhere. Applbaum could see that this mixture of moral certainty and the lure of billions of dollars in potential profits was a potent force.

"These executives seemed to believe that they are straightforwardly trying to heal the world," said Applbaum. When he was meeting them in 2000 and 2001 he had no reason to doubt these self-assessments. "They seemed to believe their products were effective and they were baffled that anyone should question their value. The pharmaceutical industry, more than other industries, can link its marketing activities to ethical objectives. The result is a marriage of the profit-seeking scheme in which disease is regarded as 'an opportunity' to the ethical view that mankind's health hangs in the balance. This helps even the most aggressive marketers trust that they are performing a public service."

Bolstering their certainty was their faith in the science behind these drugs. The fact that these SSRIs had proven clinically effective made it morally imperative that they be introduced into other cultures. The drug companies were replacing what one executive referred to as "junk science" in Japan with "first world medicine."

During his talks with the executives, consultants, and marketers for the drug companies, Applbaum heard a repeated theme. These men and women kept talking about different cultures as if they were at different stages of a predetermined evolution. The American market, with its the brand recognition, high rates of prescriptions (by specialists and nonspecialists alike), and free market pricing, was seen as the most modern and advanced of markets. Japan was fifteen years behind the United States, executives would say. Or China was five years behind Japan. The lucrative U.S. market, Applbaum could see, was the standard against which all others were measured. We were the most "evolved" culture and, as one executive said to Applbaum, their job was to "speed the evolution along," that is, to move other countries along the path to be like us.

This talk of evolutionary process wasn't idle chatter, for it was often the same executives and marketing specialists who went from country to country waiting for the right moment to make their push. "Pharmaceutical manufacturers . . . circulate internal instructional materials regarding experiences with the same product in what they consider similar markets," Applbaum said. "Managers fly about the world to training conferences where such archetypes are hardened. And old advertisements and communications strategies from the earlier stage of more 'advanced' markets are imported." With each new implementation of the mega-marketing campaign, these drug companies learned new maneuvers and strategies. They got better at helping along the evolution.

The reasons these executives were so open about this endeavor goes back to their shared belief that the evolution in question was toward higher quality science. Westerners may have lost their sense of moral authority in many areas of human endeavor, but we can still get our blood up defending our science. We lead the world in scientific discovery and medical breakthroughs, so why shouldn't the citizens of Japan and other countries around the world have access to the newest brand-name antidepressants? These molecules were created using the latest advances in science and technology. They had been reviewed by the leading researchers at the world's most famous universities and found effective in studies published in the most prestigious scientific journals. The latest antidepressants, in this moral logic, were akin to antiretrovirals, polio vaccine, and penicillin. Everyone in the world deserved access to the fruits of our scientific discoveries as a human right.

It is not an argument without merit, but it depends rather critically on the accuracy and validity of the science behind the medical advance being touted. If the science is overblown, skewed, or downright wrong, then the moral certainty that fuels the charge into other cultures becomes suspect.

Blinding Them with Science

Of all the luxuries provided him during that Glaxo-sponsored Kyoto conference in 2001, Kirmayer remembers one evening with particular relish. On the second night of the conference he was instructed to dress in a "smart suit" and was taken to the Tsuruya restaurant, one of the most exclusive and expensive restaurants in Japan. At the restaurant he was shown the guest book, where Henry Kissinger and other world leaders had left their compliments. During dinner a personal geisha sat at his arm smiling and pouring his tea and sake. After trying to make small talk with this young woman in his limited Japanese, he turned to James Ballenger to bring up a question that had been on his mind.

Ballenger was the head of the International Consensus Group on Depression. For three years he and a group of other academic researchers hosted seven meetings at various luxury resorts and hotels around the world. At these conferences, funded by Glaxo-SmithKline, Ballenger gathered prominent scholars and researchers to consider the best treatments for PTSD, panic disorder, and generalized anxiety disorder. In the end these supposedly independent scholars, with their affiliations to some of the world's finest universities, recommended that SSRIs be prescribed for all of these conditions. Tellingly, the only SSRI mentioned by name in the Consensus Group's summation paper was paroxetine, aka Paxil.

Kirmayer was curious about the relationship between the drug companies and academics like Ballenger who published the papers recommending these drugs. Wanting to be polite, he thanked Ballenger for the remarkable accommodations and treatment he was receiving. Kirmayer was, of course, in no position to take the moral high road, as he was at that very moment enjoying the splendor and luxury for which GlaxoSmithKline was picking up the tab. Nevertheless he felt compelled to ask Ballenger, as nicely as he could: Isn't this something of a conflict of interest?

Although he can't remember what Ballenger said word for word, he remembers the gist.* "He told me, 'Look, I've made my peace with this a long time ago. The drug companies are going to do this anyway—they are going to market drugs and produce guidelines, so they can either do it with input of good people who are knowledgeable and scientifically sophisticated and evenhanded or not,'" Kirmayer remembers.

"In their heart of hearts," Kirmayer said, "I think academics who have consulted with drug companies think that they are doing good and that they deserve the consulting fees and perks." In short, no

---

*Ballenger did not return phone calls requesting an interview for this book.

one seemed to be losing any sleep over the ethics of such a luxurious meeting being sponsored by a drug company. No doubt the thread count in the sheets helped in this regard.

At the time Ballenger's response did not seem unreasonable to Kirmayer. This was before it was revealed that many of the most influential studies on SSRIs, supposedly written by prominent academics, were in fact ghostwritten by private firms hired by drug companies. This was before it was widely known that many academics had taken hundreds of thousands of dollars (sometimes millions) in consulting and speaking fees while at the same time helping to hide or disguise negative data on the very drugs they were supposedly evaluating.

It has been only in the past few years, in fact, that these issues have become a public scandal prompting ongoing litigation and an investigation in the U.S. Senate. Many drugs and companies have been implicated in this recent upheaval, but one company and one drug have been at the very heart of the scandal: GlaxoSmithKline and Paxil.

Under even the mildest scrutiny, the confident marketing messages proclaiming the scientific validity of SSRIs begin to break down. Take for instance the idea, often repeated in the ads and promotional material surrounding the launch of SSRIs in Japan, that a depletion of serotonin is the root cause of depression and that SSRIs reestablish the "balance" of the "natural" chemicals in the brain. Pharmaceutical companies have been repeating this idea ever since SSRIs came on the market twenty years ago. On their website the makers of the SSRI Lexapro are still telling the story: "The naturally occurring chemical serotonin is sent from one nerve cell to the next. . . . In people with depression and anxiety, there is an imbalance of serotonin—too much serotonin is reabsorbed by the first nerve cell, so the next cell does not have enough; as in a conversation, one person might do all the talking and the other person does not get to comment, leading to a communication imbalance."

Here's how GlaxoSmithKline describes the same idea on its website advertising Paxil CR: "Normally, a chemical neurotransmitter in your brain, called serotonin, helps send messages from one brain cell to another. This is how the cells in your brain communicate. Serotonin works to keep the messages moving smoothly. However, if serotonin levels become unbalanced, communication may become disrupted and lead to depression. . . . Paxil CR helps maintain a balance of serotonin levels."

As often repeated as this story is, it turns out that there is currently no scientific consensus that depression is linked to serotonin deficiency or that SSRIs restore the brain's normal "balance" of this neurotransmitter. The idea that depression is due to deficits of serotonin was first proposed by George Ashcroft in the 1950s, when he thought he detected low levels in the brains of suicide victims and in the spinal fluid of depressed patients. Later studies, however, performed with more sensitive equipment and measures, showed no lower levels of serotonin in these populations. By 1970 Ashcroft had publicly given up on the serotonin-depression connections. To date, no lower levels of serotonin or "imbalance" of the neurotransmitter have been demonstrated in depressed patients. The American Psychiatric Press *Textbook of Clinical Psychiatry* states simply, "Additional experience has not confirmed the monoamine [of which serotonin is a subgroup] depletion hypothesis."

SSRIs don't bring a patient's brain chemistry back into balance, but rather broadly alter brain chemistry. Although that change may sometimes help a depressed patient, the idea that SSRIs restore a natural balance of serotonin is a theory without evidence. Put another way, this idea is more of a culturally shared story than a scientific fact, in the exact same way neurasthenia's invocation of "frayed nerves" was a story.

What made this story so popular was that it turned out to be an effective marketing line, first employed in the United States and Europe and then around the world. SSRIs came on the heels of the public scandal about the overprescribing of benzodiazepines. These drugs, including Valium and Librium, were initially embraced by the medical establishment until they were revealed to be highly addictive. As SSRIs came to market, the public was understandably wary of psychopharmacological agents. The story that SSRIs only helped balance natural chemicals in the brain, therefore, was just what the public needed to hear. This marketing line was useful in a similar way in Japan, where many considered Western psychiatric medicines to be harsh and unnatural.

In the end, to judge the value of a drug, its benefits must be considered in light of its risks. Unfortunately, in judging the benefit-risk balance of SSRIs one immediately runs into an even more complicated and thorny question: To what extent can the Western scientific literature describing the risks and benefits of these drugs be trusted? What worries many researchers is that the makers of pharmaceutical drugs such as SSRIs have gained remarkable control over the creation and presentation of the scientific data that purport to show that these drugs are safe and effective.

No man has fought harder to expose the process by which pharmaceutical makers control the knowledge pipeline behind their drugs than David Healy, a psychiatrist in the North Wales Department of Psychological Medicine and a professor at the University of Cardiff. Healy's particular crusade is not against SSRIs or the use of any drug in particular, but for the full and unbiased accounting of the data.* Because GlaxoSmithKline and other drug companies

---

*In the debate over the risks and benefits of SSRIs there are few people in the middle ground and a wealth of easily accessible information designed to appear

have control over the creation of the science, Healy argues, "there is almost no possibility of discrepant data emerging to trigger a thought that might be unwelcome to the marketing department of a pharmaceutical company."

This skewing and shaping of the data becomes more confounding as the information gets transmitted across cultures and languages by the marketers intent on selling the medication.

According to Healy, drug companies first started ghostwriting scientific papers for university researchers in the 1950s. Back then it was seen as a marginally disreputable practice, and these papers usually appeared only in obscure journals with little prestige or influence. But by the 1970s the drug companies had taken control of funding the major randomized control studies, and by the mid-1990s, Healy estimates, over half of the studies in the most prestigious journals were being drafted not by the university researchers supposedly heading the studies but by medical writing companies paid by the drug companies.

Once this became an accepted practice, the drug companies found that they not only had control over what information made it into print but they also had remarkable power over which university researchers rose to become stars in their field. "In effect," writes Nassir Ghaemi, director of the Mood Disorders and Psychopharmacology Programs at Tufts Medical Center, "ghost authorship is the steroid problem of academia; some of our experts get their fame

---

evenhanded that is, in fact, secretly produced by the drug companies or the most extreme critics. For instance, both the drug companies and Scientologists (who believe psychiatric drugs are basically poison) sponsor websites that appear to the reader to be created by patient advocates or impartial experts in mental health. Although the SSRI makers have actively tried to portray Healy as a man of radical opinions, the facts of Healy's professional life speak for themselves. Not only was he the former secretary of the British Association of Psychopharmacology and a professor in psychological medicine at Cardiff University, but in his medical practice he continues to use antidepressants with patients who he believes can benefit from the drugs.

artificially, their achievements appearing greater than they really are." Those who take the high ground and refuse to be part of this process run the risk of falling behind their colleagues who are, so to speak, on the juice.

In the scientific and public discussion that surrounds these drugs, it is usually only the published results that influence opinion. Unfortunately, negative results almost never see print and therefore rarely become part of the debate. A recent review of seventy-four studies of antidepressants found that nearly all (thirty-seven out of thirty-eight) of the positive studies were published in professional journals. Of the thirty-six negative studies, only three managed to make it to print. The other thirty-three negative studies either went unpublished or were reported in a form that claimed a positive outcome different from the one the study intended to examine.*

When the raw data from the published and unpublished studies are examined together, the SSRIs begin to look nothing like the miracle drug being promoted in Japan and elsewhere. An analysis of the clinical trial data submitted to the U.S. Food and Drug Administration shows that about five out of ten test subjects given an SSRI improve over a couple of weeks on the depression rating scale. This at first seems like a fantastic outcome, until one considers the placebo group, those people in the trial who were given a sugar pill. On average, four out of ten patients taking a fake pill improve. Indeed, in many of the unpublished studies, SSRIs have failed to outperform placebos.

This means that only one in ten test subjects shows a positive response that can be attributed to the effect of the SSRI. This is hardly impressive, especially when one considers the fact that "improvement" doesn't mean that the depression goes away but

---

*Searching for some secondary positive aspect in otherwise negative data is referred to as "data torturing" and is often criticized as being the statistical equivalent of placing the target after throwing the darts.

often only indicates a change on a symptom rating scale. A person who is still depressed but sleeping better, for instance, might be seen as improved. Indeed with enough test subjects, even minor changes in one or two of the checklist items can appear to be significant.

This rather anemic level of effectiveness would certainly surprise many Japanese who have been subject to the mega-marketing campaign promoting SSRIs as a cure for depression. Negative data get weeded out or spun, while even small beneficial results zoom through the supposedly scientific gatekeepers (the academics "authoring" the studies and the journal editors) to the salespeople, the marketers, and the public relations firms and out of the mouths of credulous journalists. Each stage of the process by which this information is manufactured distances the doctor and the depressed patient from the actual benefits and risks of the drug. When this information pipeline crosses cultural boundaries under the auspices of a mega-marketing campaign funded by the drug maker, the relation between the consumer's perception of the product and the science behind the drug becomes all but illusory.

In judging just how honest drug companies are being with the data, one example stands out. In July 2001, just as Glaxo-SmithKline's marketing campaign in Japan was ramping up, a paper titled "Efficacy of Paroxetine [Paxil] in the Treatment of Adolescent Major Depression: A Randomized, Controlled Trial" was published in the *Journal of the American Academy of Child and Adolescent Psychiatry,* the most influential journal in the field. Among the half dozen authors were many prominent names, including lead author Dr. Martin Keller, the chairman of psychiatry at Brown University. The study had been conducted between 1994 and 1997 and included almost three hundred depressed adolescents. It was a double-blind study—the gold standard—meaning that neither the patient nor the doctor giving the pills knew which of the subjects were getting the drug being tested rather than the placebo. In the paper the authors gave their hearty approval, writing that Paxil was "generally well tolerated and effective for major depression in adolescents."

Within a month of the publication of the study, the company sales reps were alerted to the good news. A memo dated August 2001 from Paxil Product Management to "all sales representatives selling Paxil" trumpeted "this 'cutting edge,' landmark study" as having "demonstrated REMARKABLE Efficacy and Safety in the treatment of adolescent depression."

Internal company documents that have come to light through lawsuits and government investigations report remarkably different results. Those internal memos suggest that the study had in fact failed to show a significant difference between Paxil and the placebo on any of the eight measures the study had set out to use. A company memo reported that the results had proven "insufficiently robust" and recommended that the company "effectively manage the dissemination of these data in order to minimize any potential commercial impact." The memo went on: "It would be commercially unacceptable to include a statement that efficacy had not been demonstrated, as this would undermine the profile of paroxetine (aka Paxil)."

Needless to say, this in-house assessment by GlaxoSmithKline staff stands in remarkable contrast to the published conclusion that Paxil was "well tolerated and effective for major depression in adolescents." But more disturbing still is that the published study apparently downplayed or hid the drug's side effects. Early drafts of the study, which came to light during lawsuits, show that serious side effects (including hospitalizations and suicide attempts) were more than five times more likely in the teens taking Paxil than in those taking the placebo. In addition, severe and often incapacitating problems with the nervous system were four times more likely for those on the drug. Nevertheless, in the first version of the study submitted for publication there was no mention of any serious adverse side effects. In a subsequent version there was a sentence suggesting that "worsening depression, emotional lability, headache, and hostility" were possible side effects. Even that acknowledgment was left out of the final published version of the paper that reports the side effects as only one "headache."

So here is an example of the knowledge pipeline created by GlaxoSmithKline. From the company's own internal documents we see that the study data that entered the pipeline showed that the effect of the drug on depression in teens was "insufficiently robust" and that some of those teens on the drug showed dramatic increases in hospitalizations and suicide attempts over those given the placebo. At the other end of the pipeline comes the marketing claim that the study "demonstrated **REMARKABLE** Efficacy and Safety."

The story of this study, and the problem that it highlights, is not isolated. After two decades of working at the esteemed *New England Journal of Medicine*, Dr. Marcia Angell became convinced that the system by which these drugs gain scientific status is broken. "It is simply no longer possible to believe much of the clinical research that is published, or to rely on the judgment of trusted physicians or authoritative medical guidelines," she wrote in 2009 in the *New York Review of Books*. The problems of ghostwriting and payments to researchers from the drug companies have, she said, reached their most florid form in the field of psychiatry and the studies of SSRIs.* The science behind SSRIs used to justify their sale in other cultures has proven to be suspect at best.

---

*In defending her members against Angell's charges, Dr. Nada Stotland, president of the American Psychiatric Association, replied to Angell's criticism, "It is unfair to suggest physicians are 'corrupt' for activities that were virtually universal when they occurred.'" Such a sentence can stop one cold. Is the president of the APA really falling back on that old chestnut of an excuse for bad behavior, "Everyone was doing it"? And what definition of corruption is she relying on that ensures that those in the majority cannot be at fault?

Suicides and SSRIs

The question of whether these drugs can, in some patients, increase thoughts of suicide has become a contentious public debate. Given that GlaxoSmithKline was leveraging the suicide-depression connection to sell Paxil in Japan, this question becomes even more salient. Healy estimates that SSRI trials, when taken together, show that about one in twenty patients become extremely agitated on these drugs. For some, that agitation will be so disquieting that it will spark suicidal thoughts or behavior. The likelihood is that these drugs are ineffective in most patients, work well for a small percentage of patients, and spark suicidal thoughts or behaviors in another small segment. Two well-designed studies conducted fifteen years apart both point to this conclusion. In 1993 three researchers from the Department of Psychiatry at Harvard concluded that antidepressants, including the SSRI Prozac, likely lessened the chances of suicide in some patients while raising it in others. "These observations suggest that antidepressants may redistribute the risk, attenuating risk in some patients who respond well, while possibly enhancing risk in others who respond more poorly."

Fully fifteen years later another set of researchers, these from the College of Physicians and Surgeons of Columbia University, came to a similar but more refined conclusion. This study looked closely at two years' worth of patient data and found that in adults there was no significant difference between the group that got the drug and the group that didn't. In teenagers and children, however, those who took the drug were significantly more likely than those who didn't to attempt suicide within four months after being started on the drug. Looking at the data further, researchers found one group in which the drug had a protective effect against suicidal behavior: adult men. The redistribution of the risk, in this case, appeared to be away from adult males and toward teenagers and children.

In the end it is possible that both the critics of SSRIs and their promoters might have legitimate points on the suicide question. The agitation and aggression sometimes noted in association with these drugs are most pronounced early in the treatment, the very period often focused on in clinical trials. In real-world use such negative reactions to the drug may lessen or disappear after this early period. In addition, attentive doctors may quickly take a patient off the drug, so that only patients who respond well (or at least don't spiral into suicidal behavior) continue taking the drug. Thus it is possible that these drugs increase suicidality in test subjects in short-term clinical trials, as critics have contended, *and yet*, when judged over years, reduce suicide in the overall population.

Even if it proves to be true that SSRIs reduce suicidality in large populations, the drug companies and the researchers who helped them distort or underreport negative data might still be culpable. Had those early treatment risks been accurately reported in the published research on these drugs, doctors would have had a chance to change the way they monitored their patients and been better prepared to spot a patient having a bad reaction. Because suicidal behavior has been demonstrated even in healthy subjects (those taking the drug with no symptoms of depression), doctors almost certainly would have second-guessed prescribing this medication to those with only mild symptoms of depression.

The timing of who knew what and when regarding the risks associated with Paxil is a critical issue because Japan was so late in adopting the drug. Was GlaxoSmithKline hiding or downplaying side-effect risks at the same time it was rolling out its mega-marketing campaign in Japan? Internal company documents that surfaced in a recent lawsuit appear to answer that question quite clearly. Data originally submitted to the U.S. Food and Drug Administration back in the late 1980s and early 1990s, but never published, appear to have been presented to intentionally hide results that test subjects on the drug had an eightfold increase in the risk of suicidality. "It looks like GlaxoSmithKline bamboozled the FDA," Senator Charles Grassley said in a speech on the floor of the Senate after he examined the evidence. "We cannot live in a nation where drug companies are less than candid, hide information and attempt to mislead the FDA and the public."

The extent to which the SSRI makers have manufactured and systematically controlled the creation, flow, and international distribution of the science is hard to overstate. Take a step back and look at the system as a whole, and you can suddenly see it in a different light, as a massive interconnected marketing system. Applbaum, the anthropologist who documented the SSRI invasion of Japan, puts it this way:

> Actors traditionally found outside the "distribution channel" of the market are now incorporated into it as active proponents of exchange. Physicians, academic opinion leaders, patient advocacy groups and other grass roots movements, nongovernmental organizations, public health bodies, and even ethics overseers, through one means or another, have one by one been enlisted as vehicles in the distribution chain. . . .
>
> In our pursuit of the near-utopian promise of perfect health, we have, without realizing it, given corporate marketers free rein to take control of the true instruments of our freedom: objectivity in science, ethics and fairness in health care, and the privilege to endow medicine with the autonomy to fulfill its oath to work for the benefit of the sick.

Even the patient, often now referred to as the "consumer," has been enlisted in the distribution chain. In marketing directly to the consumer through the Internet and various other avenues, drug companies can claim to be treating patients as informed consumers. Such informed consumers can be enlisted to petition their doctors and drug review boards for access to the drugs. This has been heralded as a positive change: no longer is the patient a passive recipient of the doctor's privileged knowledge. Unfortunately, the patients, particularly those living outside the United States, are often the last to know that the knowledge they are acquiring may have been manipulated to create specific beliefs and desires.

Early Adopters Have Second Thoughts

There is no doubt that the efforts of GlaxoSmithKline in Japan proved profitable. In just the first year on the market Paxil sales brought in over 100 million dollars. At the end of 2002 the company reported, "Sales of Seroxat/Paxil, GSK's leading product for depression and anxiety disorders, was the driver of growth in the CNS (Central Nervous System) therapy area, with sales of 3.1 billion, up 15% globally and 18% in the USA. International Sales of Paxil Grew 27% to $401 million led by continued strong growth in Japan, where the product was launched only two years ago." By 2008 sales of Paxil were over one billion dollars per year in Japan.

Kitanaka has been stunned to see how fast things have changed in Japan since SSRIs were introduced. "The whole culture surrounding psychiatry has changed drastically," she told me. "From a stigmatizing notion that no one talked about, depression has become one of the top concerns of people. It has become a legitimate disease at so many different levels and at the same time these changes have transformed the nature of depression as an experience itself."

Some Japanese psychiatrists, even Ono and Tajima, whom the company feted in 2000, felt they were not leading this new trend but reacting to it. Ono reports that starting in 2001 he suddenly had a rush of patients showing up at his office with either a magazine article or an advertisement in hand and wanting to talk about their depression. It was clear to him that the mild symptoms these patients described would not previously have been considered an illness. As more and more Japanese began to identify themselves as depressed and as the risks of SSRIs came to his attention, he has wondered if there were ways to reverse the trend.

"The marketing campaign has been in many ways too successful. The slogan, depression is like a 'cold of the soul,' has convinced far too many people to seek medical treatment for something that is often not an illness," Ono told me. "Perhaps we could start saying that depression is like a 'cancer of the soul.' That would be more accurate and perhaps not so many people would be willing to adopt that belief."

Dr. Tajima has come even further in his thinking. Tajima is the prominent psychiatrist who made such encouraging remarks in Kyoto in 2000 about the adoption of international diagnostic standards that would "facilitate accurate diagnosis." At the time he welcomed the introduction of SSRIs, saying that they would "contribute to reducing the burden of depression and anxiety disorders in Japanese society." For several years after the conference, Tajima was a central figure in the company's attempt to win over other psychiatrists in Japan. He was paid well by GlaxoSmithKline to give speeches and appear at conferences. The paper based on his talk at the Kyoto conference was widely used in the company's educational material.

But in the past few years he has become concerned as he's watched just how many of his countrymen have been diagnosed with depression and started on Paxil. Revelations made public by

David Healy and others have caused him to become skeptical as to whether GlaxoSmithKline has accurately reported the scientific data regarding the drug's effectiveness and risks. He has taken it upon himself to translate one of Healy's books into Japanese and now jokes that he is going to become "the David Healy of Japan."

In discussing the remarkable changes that he's seen in Japan over the past ten years, Tajima does not come off as a man who is angry with GlaxoSmithKline. Indeed, in recounting his own participation in these changes, he often laughs heartily, like a man telling the story of how he was thoroughly fooled by a talented magician or card shark. His laughter communicates "I have only myself to blame."

He maintains that Paxil is helpful for some anxiety disorders and can be used in serious cases of depression so long as the patient is monitored closely through the early days of treatment. However, he has come to believe that the drug is massively overprescribed and that it can sometimes spark suicidal thoughts in patients. "After the Ministry of Health in Japan issued a warning of a suicide risk with this drug for patients under twenty-five, many doctors and patients are now aware of this risk," says Tajima. What he can't understand, however, is why the drug remains so widely prescribed for patients with depressive symptoms that are transient and relatively mild. The warning about the risk of suicide seemed not to have had much effect against the forces of the mega-marketing campaign sponsored by GlaxoSmithKline in the years since 2000.

Tajima has also come to mistrust the confident science presented by the pharmaceutical manufacturers. Although he is aware that the drug companies don't take kindly to criticism, he is committed to fighting the good fight and getting the best information to the Japanese people any way he can.

Did he have any hope, I asked him, of challenging the imported ideas that helped popularize depression in Japan? "The force of this tide is still very strong," Tajima said. He did point to some signs that might indicate a lessening of the momentum. The marginal effectiveness of the drug has not gone unnoticed. "There are so many patients in Japan who have not improved and not recovered," he told me. "Many ordinary people now have questions about these so-called magic drugs."

As journalists often do, I saved the most uncomfortable question for the very end of my interview with Dr. Tajima. I told him that I did not want to pry too far into his personal finances, but I wanted to know how he felt about the money he had taken from GlaxoSmithKline over the years. "Yes," he said, laughing again. "This is a very important question. Some people say that this relationship between the researchers and the drug companies is a kind of prostitution. I agree. But I am not a puritan. I am a very realistic man. This is very problematic. We have to change the current situation not only in Japan but also in the United States and other countries. The strong force of the pharmaceutical industry threatens to turn medicine into a pseudoscience in the same way they have made opinion leaders in the field of Japanese psychiatry into a type of prostitute."

Then he paused, laughed again, and added, "We were very cheap prostitutes."

Conclusion

The Global Economic Crisis
and the Future of Mental Illness

Cultures become particularly vulnerable to new beliefs about the mind and madness during times of social anxiety or discord. It is no surprise that the Western form of anorexia was able to worm its way into the unconscious minds of young Hong Kong women in the uneasy years between the Tiananmen Square massacre and the British handover of the province to China. As demonstrated in Sri Lanka, the Western notion of PTSD often gains a hold because it is deployed in populations that are disoriented and reeling from wars or natural disasters. It is also no coincidence that the GlaxoSmithKline version of depression caught hold in Japan during that country's lengthy and painful recession. Ongoing economic upheaval can be particularly unsettling because the unrelenting threat to one's status, security, and future seems to come from everywhere and nowhere at the same time.

In early 2009, as I was researching the chapter on depression and Japan, the world economy went into a tailspin. What happened to the Nikkei in 1990 appeared to be happening to every major stock index, from the S&P 500 to the OMX Copenhagen 20. The globalization of the world economy, which had wrought a great many disorienting changes, had now brought us something new: a truly global economic crisis. The social upheaval that made Japan vulnerable to GlaxoSmithKline's mega-marketing campaigns was now prevalent in pretty much every country in the world.

As the crisis grew I listened for the first mental health experts to step forward with warnings about the psychological consequences of the crisis. Quick on their heels, I was sure, would come the promise of new medicines and perhaps even a new category of mental illness to explain our distress.

I didn't have to wait long.

In early February articles about the downturn's effect on mental health began to appear in major publications. "Suicides: Watching for a Recession Spike" was one headline at *Time* magazine. "Suicide experts say there is a strong correlation between acute financial strains and depression," the article reported. Near the same time, *USA Today* reported, "Signs abound that the battered economy is causing serious damage to mental health. . . . Nearly half of Americans said they were more stressed than a year ago, and about one third rated their stress level as 'extreme' in surveys conducted by the American Psychological Association."

The *New York Times* soon had its own front-page story: "Recession Anxiety Seeps into Everyday Lives." Quoting experts and individuals, the article listed over two dozen mental health problems caused by economic worries. These symptoms ranged from the mundane (sleeplessness, anxiety, constant worrying) to the severe and sometimes bizarre (struggling to breathe, rapid heartbeat, chills, choking sensation, numbness and tingling in the fingers, and arthritis). Such a wide-ranging list of potential symptoms suggested that we were in the midst of creating the symptom pool for the current economic crisis. We were publicly debating, as a culture, which symptoms and pathologies we would jointly recognize as legitimate expressions of economic anxiety.

Many of these articles pointed out that our national mental health was already poor and was now certain to get worse. The National Institute of Mental Health announced that one in every four Americans age 18 and older suffers from a diagnosable mental disorder *each year*. Among young adults mental illnesses had become the leading cause of disability. There were other troubling signs: a study came out suggesting that the mental disorders sparked by Hurricane Katrina were proving strangely resistant to both treatment and the healing effect of time; fully three years after the fact, the incidence of mood disorders and PTSD linked to the disaster was still rising in Louisiana.

To counter such bad news, Senior Vice President Ken Johnson of the pharmaceutical advocacy group PhRMA announced that no fewer than 301 new medicines were in development to treat mental illnesses, including sixty-six for depression and fifty-four for anxiety disorders. It was important, given the worrisome trends, that the public knew that new medications were on the way to help people "live longer, happier, healthier lives."*

Of course, just what types of disorders those 301 new drugs will be tasked to treat depends largely on the American Psychiatric Association, which will soon publish a new edition of its influential diagnostic manual, the *DSM-V*. The research journals have been filled with suggestions for changes and additions and APA work groups are currently in the process of hashing out which disorders will be included, changed, or cut.

As if to demonstrate the point that the creation of mental illness categories remains as much a social and cultural endeavor as a scien-

---

*In the same release, PhRMA announced that it had helped launch a new consumer advocacy site featuring the well-known actor from *The Sopranos*, Joe Pantoliano, who had publicly admitted to struggling with depression. "The goal," according to the No Kidding, Me Too website, was to "make brain disease cool and sexy."

tific process, the APA is soliciting input from the public. As of this writing there is still a "Make a Suggestion" link on the association's website describing the *DSM-V* project. Click on that link and you are presented with a number of options, including "Submit suggestions for deletion of an existing disorder" and "Submit suggestions for a new disorder to be considered for addition to *DSM-V*." All suggestions, the public is promised, will be routed to the proper *DSM-V* work group for debate.

If I had to lay a bet on which new disorder recently discussed in the psychiatric literature has the most promising future, it would be "post-traumatic embitterment disorder." PTED describes the reaction to an exceptionally negative but not life-threatening event, such as conflict in the workplace, sudden unemployment, the loss of social status, and separation from one's social group. Symptoms include embitterment, feelings of injustice, and helplessness.

If PTED can get enough allies on the right *DSM-V* work groups and a multinational drug company with a new drug targeting the condition, this disorder has the chance to be the next PTSD, for it seems well suited to describe many of the reactions to the precipitous cultural changes during this time of globalization and economic crisis. Indeed the disorder was first "discovered" among East Germans who had become unmoored, unemployed, and insecure in the social upheaval following the fall of the Berlin Wall.

Whatever new disorders end up in the *DSM-V* and whatever new drugs and treatments are declared scientifically proven to be effective for treating them, there is no doubt that the American public will show intense interest. We are a psychologically oriented people. Experts will appear on talk shows and provide quotes and commentary for journalists. Over time these new discoveries will become cultural certainties, conventional wisdom. In this process these new disorders will further shape our conscious and unconscious senses of self.

Then the Western mental health profession will take the show on the road. At international conferences in exotic locales professionals will train foreign healers in these new disease categories. Drug companies lured by potential profits will engage in ever more sophisticated mega-marketing campaigns. In cultures made vulnerable by the global financial crisis and the speed of social change, the seeds of these ideas will no doubt find fertile ground.

If the irony isn't already obvious, let me make it clear: offering the latest Western mental health theories in an attempt to ameliorate the psychological stress caused by globalization is not a solution; *it is a part of the problem.* By undermining both local beliefs about healing and culturally created conceptions of the self, we are speeding along the disorienting changes that are at the very heart of much of the world's mental distress. It is the psychiatric equivalent of handing out blankets to sick natives without considering the pathogens that hide deep in the fabric.

While I was in Zanzibar researching how Swahili beliefs were mixing with Western biomedical notions of mental illness, my wife, who is a psychiatrist, sent me a text message from our home in San Francisco. The brief note told of a tough day. A patient in her private practice had suffered a psychotic break and had to be admitted to a psychiatric ward.

The note reminded me of a point my wife had made often: while I was traveling the world documenting how Western-born cultural currents are altering beliefs about the mind, mental health professionals in the United States and elsewhere had little choice but to do the best they could with the knowledge and technology they had at hand. She worried, you see, that this book would unfairly disparage the mental health profession, a group of people, including herself, who are doing their best to heal troubled minds.

Keeping that concern in mind, I have tried to avoid making the clichéd argument that other, more traditional cultures necessarily have it right when it comes to treating mental illness. All cultures struggle with these intractable diseases with varying degrees of compassion and cruelty, equanimity and fear. My point is not that they necessarily have it right—only that they have it different.

It is not surprising that we want to believe everyone is just like us. As with any generation in human history, we have little awareness of how our culture shapes our mental life because it so envelops us, informing both our conscious and our unconscious thinking. We are like swimmers out of sight of land: it is difficult to gauge the direction and strength of the cultural current that carries us along. Difficult, certainly, but not impossible. As this book suggests, deep explorations into the beliefs of other cultures can reveal our own cultural biases in startling ways.

So what does a cross-cultural perspective reveal about our conception of the mind?

The ideas we export to other cultures often have at their heart a particularly American brand of hyperintrospection and hyperindividualism. These beliefs remain deeply influenced by the Cartesian split between the mind and the body, the Freudian duality between the conscious and unconscious, as well as teeming numbers of self-help philosophies and schools of therapy that have encouraged us to separate the health of the individual from the health of the group. Even the fascinating biomedical scientific research into the workings of the brain has, on a cultural level, further removed our understanding of the mind from the social and natural world it navigates. On its website advertising its antidepressant, one drug company illustrates how far this reductive thinking has gone: "Just as a cake recipe requires you to use flour, sugar, and baking powder in the right amounts, your brain needs a fine chemical balance in order to perform at its best." The Western mind, endlessly parsed by generations of philosophers, theorists, and researchers, has now been reduced to a batter of chemicals we carry around in the mixing bowl of our skulls.

What is certain is that in other places in the world, cultural conceptions of the mind remain more intertwined with a variety of religious and cultural beliefs as well as the ecological and social world. They have not yet separated the mind from the body, nor have they disconnected individual mental health from that of the group.

With little appreciation of these differences, we continue our efforts to convince the rest of the world to think like us. Given the level of contentment and psychological health our cultural beliefs about the mind have brought us, perhaps it's time that we rethink our generosity.

Sources

Introduction

American Psychiatric Association. (1994). *DSM-IV: Diagnostic and Statistical Manual of Mental Disorders, Fourth Edition.*

Hacking, I. (2002). *Mad Travelers: Reflections on the Reality of Transient Mental Illnesses.* Harvard University Press.

Okasha, A. (1999). Mental Health in the Middle East: An Egyptian Perspective. *Clinical Psychology Review,* 19 (8), 917–933.

Chapter 1
The Rise of Anorexia in Hong Kong

This chapter relied heavily on the work and generosity of Sing Lee and his assistant, Jenny Ng. Lee's willingness to arrange interviews with his patients and his introduction to other experts in Hong Kong and elsewhere were beyond the call of duty. I am grateful also for the honesty and openness of the patients who spoke with me. For those interested in diving into this subject further I highly recommend the Lee papers listed below. They are remarkably readable and deeply philosophical contemplations on the connection between culture and mental illness. They should some day be collected under one cover. Edward Shorter's historical work on anorexia, hysteria, and the nature of psychosomatic illnesses informed both this chapter and some key ideas that play out through the book.

Here is a list of the papers and books that also were helpful:

Aderibigbe, Y. A., & Pandurangi, A. K. (1995). The Neglect of Culture in Psychiatric Nosology: The Case of Culture Bound Syndromes. *International Journal of Social Psychiatry,* 41(4), 235.

American Psychiatric Association. (2000). *DSM-IV-TR: Diagnostic and Statistical Manual of Mental Disorders, Fourth Edition (Text Revision)* (p. 943).

Andepson-Fye, E. P. (2003). Never Leave Yourself: Ethnopsychology as Mediator of Psychological Globalization among Belizean Schoolgirls. *Ethos,* 31(1), 59–94.

Arnett, J. J. (1999). Adolescent Storm and Stress, Reconsidered. *American Psychologist,* 54(5), 317–326.

———. (2002). The Psychology of Globalization. *American Psychologist,* 57(10), 774–783.

———. (2003). *Adolescence and Emerging Adulthood: A Cultural Approach.* Prentice Hall.

Baer, M. (1992). *Theatre and Disorder in Late Georgian London.* Clarendon Press.

Banks, C. G. (1992). "Culture" in Culture-Bound Syndromes: The Case of Anorexia Nervosa. *Social Science & Medicine,* 34(8), 867.

———. (1996). "There Is No Fat in Heaven": Religious Asceticism and the Meaning of Anorexia Nervosa. *Ethos,* 24(1), 107–135.

Becker, A. E. (2004a). New Global Perspectives on Eating Disorders. *Culture, Medicine and Psychiatry,* 28(4), 433–437.

———. (2004b). Television, Disordered Eating, and Young Women in Fiji: Negotiating Body Image and Identity During Rapid Social Change. *Culture, Medicine and Psychiatry,* 28(4), 533–559.

———. (2007). Culture and Eating Disorders Classification. *International Journal of Eating Disorders,* 40(53), 5111–5116.

Bishop, K. (1994, December 20). KELY to Tackle Eating Disorders. *South China Morning Post.*

Bordo, S. (1996). Anorexia Nervosa: Psychopathology as the Crystallization of Culture. In A. Garry & M. Pearsall, eds., *Women, Knowledge, and Reality. Explorations in Feminist Philosophy,* Routledge.

Bordo, S., & Heywood, L. (2003). *Unbearable Weight: Feminism, Western Culture, and the Body.* University of California Press.

Bruch, H. (1985). Four Decades of Eating Disorders. In D. M. Gardener & P. E. Garfinkel, eds., *Handbook of Psychotherapy for Anorexia Nervosa and Bulimia* (pp. 7–18).

———. (2001). *The Golden Cage: The Enigma of Anorexia Nervosa.* Harvard University Press.

Brumberg, J. J. (1988). *Fasting Girls: The Emergence of Anorexia Nervosa as a Modern Disease.* Harvard University Press.

———. (2000). *Fasting Girls: The History of Anorexia Nervosa.* Vintage Books.

———. (1998). *The Body Project: An Intimate History of American Girls.* Vintage Books.

Chan, H., & Lee, R. P. L. (1995). Hong Kong Families: At the Cross-roads of Modernism and Traditionalism. *Journal of Comparative Family Studies,* 26(1).

Chan, Z., & Ma, J. (2002). Anorexic Eating: Two Case Studies in Hong Kong. *Qualitative Report,* 7, 1–14.

Chan, Z., & Ma. J. (2003). Anorexic Body: A Qualitative Study. *Forum Qualitative Sozialforschung/Forum: Qualitative Social Research,* 4(1), Art 1.

Cheung, D. (1994, December 4). Dieting Dangers. *South China Morning Post.*

Cohen, G. L., & Prinstein, M. J. (2006). Peer Contagion of Aggression and Health Risk Behavior among Adolescent Males: An Experimental Investigation of Effects on Public Conduct and Private Attitudes. *Child Development,* 77(4), 967–983.

Cummins, L. H., Simmons, A. M., & Zane, N. W. S. (2005). Eating Disorders in Asian Populations: A Critique of Current Approaches to the Study of Culture, Ethnicity, and Eating Disorders. *American Journal of Orthopsychiatry,* 75(4), 553–574.

Dennis, C. (2004). Mental Health: Asia's Tigers Get the Blues. *Nature,* 429(6993), 696–698.

Dinicola, V. F. (1990). Anorexia Multiforme: Self-Starvation in Historical and Cultural Context, Part I: Self-Starvation as a Historical Chameleon. *Transcultural Psychiatry,* 27(3), 165.

Dishion, T. J., & Dodge, K. A. (2005). Peer Contagion in Interventions for Children and Adolescents: Moving towards an Understanding of the Ecology and Dynamics of Change. *Journal of Abnormal Child Psychology,* 33(3), 395–400.

Dolan, B. (1991). Cross-Cultural Aspects of Anorexia Nervosa and Bulimia: A Review. *International Journal of Eating Disorders,* 10(1), 67–79.

Dresser, R. (1984). Cited in J. J. Brumberg, *Fasting Girls: The History of Anorexia Nervosa.*

Garner, D. M., & Garfinkel, P. E. (1985). *Handbook of Psychotherapy for Anorexia Nervosa and Bulimia*. Guilford Press.

The Girl Who Wants to Die. (1996, November 30). *South China Morning Post*.

Gordon, R. A. (2000). *Eating Disorders: Anatomy of a Social Epidemic*. Blackwell.

Gremillion, H. (1992). Psychiatry as Social Ordering: Anorexia Nervosa, a Paradigm. *Social Science & Medicine*, 35(1), 57–71.

———. (2003). *Feeding Anorexia: Gender and Power at a Treatment Center*. Duke University Press.

Habermas, T. (1989). The Psychiatric History of Anorexia Nervosa and Bulimia Nervosa: Weight Concerns and Bulimic Symptoms in Early Case Reports. *International Journal of Eating Disorders*, 8(3), 351–359.

———. (1996). In Defense of Weight Phobia as the Central Organizing Motive in Anorexia Nervosa: Historical and Cultural Arguments for a Culture-Sensitive Psychological Conception. *International Journal of Eating Disorders*, 19(4), 317–334.

Hermans, H. J., & Dimaggio, G. (2007). Self, Identity, and Globalization in Times of Uncertainty: A Dialogical Analysis. *Review of General Psychology*, 11(1), 31.

Higginbotham, N., & Connor, L. (1989). Professional Ideology and the Construction of Western Psychiatry in Southeast Asia. *International Journal of Health Services: Planning, Administration, Evaluation*, 19(1), 63.

Hoshmand, L. T. (2003). Moral Implications of Globalization and Identity. *American Psychologist*, 58(10), 814–815.

Hsu, L. K., & Lee, S. (1993). Is Weight Phobia Always Necessary for a Diagnosis of Anorexia Nervosa? *American Journal of Psychiatry*, 150(10), 1466.

Jensen, L. A. (2003). Coming of Age in a Multicultural World: Globalization and Adolescent Cultural Identity Formation. *Applied Developmental Science*, 7(3), 189–196.

Katzman, M. A., & Lee, S. (1997). Beyond Body Image: The Integration of Feminist and Transcultural Theories in the Understanding of Self Starvation. *International Journal of Eating Disorders*, 22(4), 385–394.

Khandelwal, S. K., Sharan, P., & Saxena, S. (1995). Eating Disorders: An Indian Perspective. *International Journal of Social Psychiatry*, 41(2), 132.

Kim, U., & Park, Y. S. (2005). Integrated Analysis of Indigenous Psychologies: Comments and Extensions of Ideas Presented by Shams, Jackson, Hwang and Kashima. *Asian Journal of Social Psychology,* 8(1), 75–95.

Kleinman, A. (1999). The Moral Economy of Depression and Neurasthenia in China: A Few Comments on Sing Lee's "Diagnosis Postponed: Shenjing Shuairuo and the Transformation of Psychiatry in Post-Mao China," by Sing Lee. *Culture, Medicine and Psychiatry,* 23(3), 389–392.

Lai, K. Y. C. (2000). Anorexia Nervosa in Chinese Adolescents: Does Culture Make a Difference? *Journal of Adolescence,* 23(5), 561–568.

Lai, K. Y. C., Pang, A. H. T., & Wong, C. K. (1995). Case Study: Early-Onset Anorexia Nervosa in a Chinese Boy. *Journal of the American Academy of Child and Adolescent Psychiatry,* 34(3), 383–386.

Law, N. (2001, April 4). Eating Disorders Spread among Youth. *South China Morning Post.*

Lee, S. (1989). Anorexia Nervosa in Hong Kong. Why Not More in Chinese? *British Journal of Psychiatry,* 154(5), 683–688.

———. (1991). Anorexia Nervosa in Hong Kong: A Chinese Perspective. *Psychological Medicine,* 21(3), 703–711.

———. (1991a). Anorexia Nervosa across Cultures. *British Journal of Psychiatry,* 158, 284–285.

———. (1991b). Eating Disorder in Asian Women. *British Journal of Psychiatry,* 158(1), 131b.

———. (1992). Bulimia Nervosa in Hong Kong Chinese Patients. *British Journal of Psychiatry,* 161(4), 545–551.

———. (1993). Response to Sing Lee's Review of "Transcultural Aspects of Eating Disorders": Reply. *Transcultural Psychiatric Research Review,* 30, 296.

———. (1994a). The Diagnostic Interview Schedule and Anorexia Nervosa in Hong Kong. *Archives of General Psychiatry,* 51(3), 251–252.

———. (1994b). The Definition of Anorexia Nervosa. *British Journal of Psychiatry,* 165(6), 841.

———. (1995). Self-Starvation in Context: Towards a Culturally Sensitive Understanding of Anorexia Nervosa. *Social Science & Medicine,* 41(1), 25–36.

————. (1996). Reconsidering the Status of Anorexia Nervosa as a Western Culture-Bound Syndrome. *Social Science & Medicine,* 42(1), 21–34.

————. (1997). How Lay Is Lay? Chinese Students' Perceptions of Anorexia Nervosa in Hong Kong. *Social Science & Medicine,* 44(4), 491–502.

————. (1998a). Global Modernity and Eating Disorders in Asia. *European Eating Disorders Review,* 6(3), 151–153.

————. (1998b). Estranged Bodies, Simulated Harmony, and Misplaced Cultures: Neurasthenia in Contemporary Chinese Society. *Psychosomatic Medicine,* 60(4), 448–457.

————. (1999a). Fat, Fatigue and the Feminine: The Changing Cultural Experience of Women in Hong Kong. *Culture, Medicine and Psychiatry,* 23(1), 51–73.

————. (1999b). Diagnosis Postponed: Shenjing Shuairuo and the Transformation of Psychiatry in Post-Mao China. *Culture, Medicine and Psychiatry,* 23(3), 349–380.

————. (2001a). From Diversity to Unity: The Classification of Mental Disorders in 21st-Century China. *Psychiatric Clinics of North America,* 24(3), 421–431.

————. (2001b). Fat Phobia in Anorexia Nervosa: Whose Obsession Is It? In M. Nasser, M. Katzman, & R. A. Gordon, eds., *Eating Disorders and Cultures in Transitions,* (pp. 40–54).

————. (2002). Socio-Cultural and Global Health Perspectives for the Development of Future Psychiatric Diagnostic Systems. *Psychopathology,* 35(2–3), 152–157.

————. (2004). Engaging Culture: An Overdue Task for Eating Disorders Research. *Culture, Medicine and Psychiatry,* 28(4), 617–621.

Lee, S., Chan, Y. Y. L., & Hsu, L. K. G. (2003). The Intermediate-Term Outcome of Chinese Patients with Anorexia Nervosa in Hong Kong. *American Journal of Psychiatry,* 160(5), 967–972.

Lee, S., Chan, Y. Y., Kwok, K., & Hsu, L. K. (2005). Relationship between Control and the Intermediate Term Outcome of Anorexia Nervosa in Hong Kong. *Australian & New Zealand Journal of Psychiatry,* 39(3), 141.

Lee, S., Ho, T. P., & Hsu, L. K. G. (1993). Fat Phobic and Non–Fat Phobic Anorexia Nervosa: A Comparative Study of 70 Chinese Patients in Hong Kong. *Psychological Medicine,* 23(4), 999–1017.

Lee, S., & Kleinman, A. (2007). Are Somatoform Disorders Changing with Time? The Case of Neurasthenia in China. *Psychosomatic Medicine*, 69(9), 846.

Lee, S., Kwok, K., Liau, C., & Leung, T. (2002). Screening Chinese Patients with Eating Disorders Using the Eating Attitudes Test in Hong Kong. *International Journal of Eating Disorders*, 32(1), 91–97.

Lee, S., & Kwok, K. (2005). Cross-Cultural Perspectives on Anorexia Nervosa without Fat Phobia. In C. Norring & R. Palmer, eds., *EDNOS, Eating Disorders Not Otherwise Specified: Scientific and Clinical Perspectives on the Other Eating Disorders* (p. 204), Routledge.

Lee, S., & Lee, A. M. (2000). Disordered Eating in Three Communities of China: A Comparative Study of Female High School Students in Hong Kong, Shenzhen, and Rural Hunan. *International Journal of Eating Disorders*, 27, 317–327.

Lee, S., Lee, A. M., Ngai, E., Lee, D. T. S., & Wing, Y. K. (2001). Rationales for Food Refusal in Chinese Patients with Anorexia Nervosa. *International Journal of Eating Disorders*, 29(2), 224–229.

Lee, S., Ng, K. L., Kwok, K. P. S., & Tsang, A. (2009). Prevalence and Correlates of Social Fears in Hong Kong. *Journal of Anxiety Disorders*, 23(3), 327–332.

Lee, S., & Tsang, A. (2009). A Population-Based Study of Depression and Three Kinds of Frequent Pain Conditions and Depression in Hong Kong. *Pain Medicine*, 10(1), 155–163.

Lee, S., Tsang, A., Li, X., Phillips, M. R., & Kleinman, A. (2007). Attitudes toward Suicide among Chinese People in Hong Kong. *Suicide & Life-Threatening Behavior*, 37(5), 565–575.

Lee, S., Tsang, A., Zhang, M., Huang, Y., He, Y., Liu, Z., et al. (2007). Lifetime Prevalence and Inter-Cohort Variation in *DSM-IV* Disorders in Metropolitan China. *Psychological Medicine*, 37(1), 61–71.

Lee, S. W., Stewart, S. M., Striegel-Moore, R. H., Lee, S., Ho, S., Lee, P. W. H., et al. (2007). Validation of the Eating Disorder Diagnostic Scale for Use with Hong Kong Adolescents. *International Journal of Eating Disorders*, 40(6), 569–574.

Leung, S. K., & Lee, S. (1997). The Variable Presentation and Early Recognition of Anorexia Nervosa in Hong Kong. *Hong Kong Medical Journal*, 3, 433–435.

Lim, S. G. (2000). The Center Can(not) Hold: U.S. Women's Studies and Global Feminism. *American Studies International*, 38(8).

Littlewood, R. (1995a). Psychopathology and Personal Agency: Modernity, Culture Change and Eating Disorders in South Asian Societies. *British Journal of Medical Psychology*, 68, 45.

————. (2004). Commentary: Globalization, Culture, Body Image, and Eating Disorders. *Culture, Medicine and Psychiatry*, 28(4), 597–602.

Luk, H. (2000, June 26). Teenagers Risk Health in Quest for Beauty. *Hong Kong Mail.*

Ma, J. L. C. (2005). Family Treatment for a Chinese Family with an Adolescent Suffering from Anorexia Nervosa: A Case Study. *Family Journal*, 13(1), 19.

————. (2007). Living in Poverty: A Qualitative Inquiry of Emaciated Adolescents and Young Women Coming from Low-Income Families in a Chinese Context. *Family Social Work*, 12(2), 152–160.

Ma, J. L. C., & Chan, Z. C. Y. (2003). The Different Meanings of Food in Chinese Patients Suffering from Anorexia Nervosa: Implications for Clinical Social Work Practice. *Social Work in Mental Health*, 2(1), 47–70.

Ma, J. L. C., Chow, M. Y. M., Lee, S., & Lai, K. (2002). Family Meaning of Self-Starvation: Themes Discerned in Family Treatment in Hong Kong. *Journal of Family Therapy*, 24(1), 57.

Micale, M. (1993). On the "Disappearance" of Hysteria: A Study in the Clinical Deconstruction of a Diagnosis. *Isis*, 84(3), 496–526.

————. (1994). *Approaching Hysteria: Disease and Its Interpretations.* Princeton University Press.

Miller, M. N., & Pumariega, A. J. (2001). Culture and Eating Disorders: A Historical and Cross-Cultural Review. *Psychiatry: Interpersonal & Biological Processes*, 64(2), 93–110.

Mumford, D. (1995). From Fasting Saints to Anorexic Girls. Review of Walter Vandereycken & Ron van Deth. *European Eating Disorders Review*, 3(2), 296.

Nasser, M., Katzman, M., & Gordon, R. A. (2001). *Eating Disorders and Cultures in Transition.* Brunner-Routledge.

Ngai, E. S. W., Lee, S., & Lee, A. M. (2000). The Variability of Phenomenology in Anorexia Nervosa. *Acta Psychiatrica Scandinavia*, 102, 314–317.

Oppenheim, J., & Oppenheim, J. (1991). *"Shattered Nerves": Doctors, Patients, and Depression in Victorian England.* Oxford University Press.

Orbach, S. (1981). *Fat Is a Feminist Issue.* Pax.

Parsons, C. (1995, September 2). Girl Who Died on Street Was a Walking Skeleton. *South China Morning Post.*

Pike, K. M., & Borovoy, A. (2004). The Rise of Eating Disorders in Japan: Issues of Culture and Limitations of the Model of "Westernization." *Culture, Medicine and Psychiatry,* 28(4), 493–531.

Polinska, W. (2000). Bodies under Siege: Eating Disorders and Self-Mutilation among Women. *Journal of the American Academy of Religion,* 68(3), 569–590.

Russell, G. F. (1985). The Changing Nature of Anorexia Nervosa: An Introduction to the Conference. *Journal of Psychiatric Research,* 19 (2–3), 101.

Russell, G. F. M., & Treasure, J. (1989). The Modern History of Anorexia Nervosa: An Interpretation of Why the Illness Has Changed. *Annals of the New York Academy of Sciences,* 575, 13–30.

Shorter, E. (1985). *Bedside Manners: The Troubled History of Doctors and Patients.* Simon & Schuster.

———. (1987). The First Great Increase in Anorexia Nervosa. *Journal of Social History,* 21(1), 69–96.

———. (1992). *From Paralysis to Fatigue: A History of Psychosomatic Illness in the Modern Era.* Free Press.

———. (2008). History of Psychiatry. *Current Opinion in Psychiatry,* 21(6), 593.

Shorter, E., & Keefe, P. H. (1994). *From the Mind into the Body: The Cultural Origins of Psychosomatic Symptoms.* Free Press.

Showalter, E. (1985). *The Female Malady: Women, Madness, and English Culture, 1830–1980.* Pantheon.

Simpson, K. J. (2002). Anorexia Nervosa and Culture. *Journal of Psychiatric and Mental Health Nursing,* 9(1), 65–71.

Smith, A. (1998, March 29). Beauty Queens "Unhealthy" Slim. *South China Morning Post.*

Starved for Attention. (1997, November 26). *South China Morning Post.*

Steiger, H. (1993). Anorexia Nervosa: Is It the Syndrome or the Theorist That Is Culture- and Gender-Bound? *Transcultural Psychiatric Research Review,* 30(4), 347–358.

Swartz, L. (1987). Illness Negotiation: The Case of Eating Disorders. *Social Science & Medicine,* 24(7), 613–618.

Tang, E. (1995, July 20). Swallowing the Lies about Beauty Can Make You Sick. *The Standard* (Hong Kong).

Tseng, W. S. (2006). From Peculiar Psychiatric Disorders through Culture-Bound Syndromes to Culture-Related Specific Syndromes. *Transcultural Psychiatry,* 43(4), 554.

Tseng, W. S., & Hsu, J. (1969). Chinese Culture, Personality Formation and Mental Illness. *International Journal of Social Psychiatry,* 16(1), 5–14.

Vandereycken, W. (2006). Denial of Illness in Anorexia Nervosa: A Conceptual Review. Part 1, Diagnostic Significance and Assessment. *European Eating Disorders Review,* 14(5), 341–351.

Vandereycken, W., & Hoek, H. W. (1992). Are Eating Disorders Culture-Bound Syndromes? In K. Halmi, ed., *Psychobiology and Treatment of Anorexia Nervosa and Bulimia Nervosa* (pp. 19–36). American Psychiatric Publishing.

Weiss, M. G. (1995). Eating Disorders and Disordered Eating in Different Cultures. *Psychiatric Clinics of North America,* 18(3), 261.

Wong, B. (n.d.). Jury Delivers Open Verdict on Dead Schoolgirl. *The Standard* (Hong Kong).

Chapter 2
The Wave That Brought PTSD to Sri Lanka

I owe a great many debts on this chapter, and they go back many years. In particular I've relied on the work of Allan Young and his trenchant book *Harmony of Illusions: Inventing Post-Traumatic Stress Disorder.* Two up-and-coming scholars were particularly giving of their time: Gaithri Fernando and Alex Argenti-Pillen. It was through the analyses of these two researchers that I saw the most complex and compelling picture of the mental landscape of the Sri Lankan people. Many of my ideas about the impact of culture on conceptions of psychological trauma came from my years chronicling the recovered memory wars. My former coauthor, Richard Ofshe, as well as Paul McHugh, and Fred Crews, were excellent guides in this regard.

Here is a more extensive list of the sources:

After the Waves: Teaching and Healing. (2006). January 5 *Pennsylvania Gazette.*

Almedom, A. M., & Summerfield, D. (2004). Mental Well-Being in Settings of "Complex Emergency": An Overview. *Journal of Biosocial Science,* 36(4), 381–388.

Amarasingham, L. R. (1980). Movement among Healers in Sri Lanka: A Case Study of a Sinhalese Patient. *Culture, Medicine and Psychiatry,* 4(1), 71–92.

Amatruda, K. Tsunami Journal. www.psychceu.com/tsunami/tsunami journal.html.

———. (n.d.). A Field Guide to Disaster Mental Health: The Very Big Wave and the Mean Old Storm. www.psychceu.com/Disaster Response/field_guide.asp.

Amatruda, K., & Helm-Simpson, P. (1997). *Sandplay: The Sacred Healing. A Guide to Symbolic Process.* Phoenix Helm Simpson.

Argenti-Pillen, A. (1999). The Discourse on Trauma in Non-Western Cultural Contexts. In A. MacFarlane, R. Yehuda, & A. Shalev, eds., *International Handbook of Human Response to Trauma.* Springer.

———. (2003). *Masking Terror: How Women Contain Violence in Southern Sri Lanka.* University of Pennsylvania Press.

Armagan, E., Engindeniz, Z., Devay, A. O., Erdur, B., & Ozcakir, A. (2006). Frequency of Post-Traumatic Stress Disorder among Relief Force Workers after the Tsunami in Asia: Do Rescuers Become Victims? *Prehospital and Disaster Medicine: The Official Journal of the National Association of EMS Physicians and the World Association for Emergency and Disaster Medicine in Association with the Acute Care Foundation,* 21(3), 168–172.

Baggerly, J. (n.d.). Tsunami Relief Work in Sri Lanka: Professor Provides Play Therapy Techniques. www.coedu.usf.edu/.

Baldwin, S. A., Williams, D. C., & Houts, A. C. (2004). The Creation, Expansion, and Embodiment of Posttraumatic Stress Disorder: A Case Study in Historical Critical Psychopathology. *Scientific Review of Mental Health Practice,* 3(33–52).

Berntsen, D., & Rubin, D. C. (2008). The Reappearance Hypothesis Revisited: Recurrent Involuntary Memories after Traumatic Events and in Everyday Life. *Memory & Cognition,* 36(2), 449–460.

Bhugra, D., & van Ommeren, M. (2006). Mental Health, Psychosocial Support and the Tsunami. *International Review of Psychiatry,* 18(3), 213–216.

Bloom, S. L. (1999). Our Hearts and Our Hopes Are Turned to Peace. In A. MacFarlane, R. Yenuda, & A. Shalev, eds., *International Handbook of Human Response to Trauma.* Springer.

Bodkin, J. A., Pope, H. G., Detke, M. J., & Hudson, J. I. (2007). Is PTSD Caused by Traumatic Stress? *Journal of Anxiety Disorders,* 21(2), 176–182.

Bonanno, G. A. (2004). Loss, Trauma, and Human Resilience. *American Psychologist,* 59(1), 20–28.

Bracken, P. J. (2001). Post-Modernity and Post-Traumatic Stress Disorder. *Social Science & Medicine,* 53(6), 733–743.

Bracken, P. J., Giller, J. E., & Summerfield, D. (1995). Psychological Responses to War and Atrocity: The Limitations of Current Concepts. *Social Science & Medicine,* 40(8), 1073–1082.

Bracken, P., Giller, J. E., & Summerfield, D. (1997). Rethinking Mental Health Work with Survivors of Wartime Violence and Refugees. *Journal of Refugee Studies,* 10(4), 431–442.

Bracken, P. J., & Petty, C. (1998). *Rethinking the Trauma of War.* Free Association Books.

Breslau, J. (2000). Globalizing Disaster Trauma: Psychiatry, Science, and Culture after the Kobe Earthquake. *Ethos,* 28(2), 174–197.

Brown, D. (2000). Time Could Be the Active Ingredient in Post-Trauma Debriefing. *British Medical Journal,* 320, 942.

Bryant, R. A., & Njenga, F. G. (2006). Cultural Sensitivity: Making Trauma Assessment and Treatment Plans Culturally Relevant. *Journal of Clinical Psychiatry,* 67 Suppl. 2, 74–79.

Cameron, D. (2005, January 24). Australia to Help Tackle Depression. *The Age* (Australia).

Cantor, C. (2008). Post-Traumatic Stress Disorder's Future. *British Journal of Psychiatry: The Journal of Mental Science,* 192(5), 394; author reply 395.

Carballo, M., Heal, B., & Hernandez, M. (2005). Psychosocial Aspects of the Tsunami. *Journal of the Royal Society of Medicine,* 98, 396–399.

Carlos, O. J., & Njenga, F. G. (2006). Lessons in Posttraumatic Stress Disorder from the Past: Venezuela Floods and Nairobi Bombing. *Journal of Clinical Psychiatry,* 67, 56.

Cheng, T. (2005, January 25). Ghosts Stalk Thai Tsunami Survivors. BBC News.

Davidson, J., Baldwin, D., Stein, D. J., Kuper, E., Benattia, I., Ahmed, S., et al. (2006). Treatment of Posttraumatic Stress Disorder with Venlafaxine Extended Release: A 6-Month Randomized Controlled Trial. *Archives of General Psychiatry,* 63(10), 1158.

Davidson, J. R. (2006). Pharmacologic Treatment of Acute and Chronic Stress Following Trauma: 2006. *Journal of Clinical Psychiatry,* 67 Suppl. 2, 34–39.

Davidson, J. R. T. (2006). After the Tsunami: Mental Health Challenges to the Community for Today and Tomorrow. *Journal of Clinical Psychiatry,* 67 Suppl. 2, 3–8.

Davis, T. (2007, February 13). Honored for Tsunami Relief: Mental Health Team from N.J. Aids Sri Lanka. *The Record.* (New Jersey).

de Silva, P. (2006). The Tsunami and Its Aftermath in Sri Lanka: Explorations of a Buddhist Perspective. *International Review of Psychiatry,* 18(3), 281–287.

Devilly, G. J., & Cotton, P. (2003). Psychological Debriefing and the Workplace: Defining a Concept, Controversies and Guidelines for Intervention. *Australian Psychologist,* 38(2), 144–150.

Devilly, G. J., & Cotton, P. (2004). Caveat Emptor, Caveat Venditor, and Critical Incident Stress Debriefing/Management (CISD/M). *Australian Psychologist,* 39(1), 35–40.

Devilly, G. J., Gist, R., & Cotton, P. (2006). Ready! Fire! Aim! The Status of Psychological Debriefing and Therapeutic Interventions: In the Work Place and after Disasters. *Review of General Psychology,* 10(4), 318.

Doherty, K. (2007, September 4). Tsunami Prompts Sri Lanka to Tackle Mental Health. Reuters.

Eisenbruch, M. (1984). Cross-Cultural Aspects of Bereavement. I: A Conceptual Framework for Comparative Analysis. *Culture, Medicine and Psychiatry,* 8(3), 283–309.

Faculty. (2005, January 5). Responding to the Aftermath of the Tsunami: Counseling with Caution. Press Release. University of Colombo, Sri Lanka.

Fernando, G. A. (2004). Working with Survivors of War in Non-Western Cultures: The Role of the Clinical Psychologist. *Intervention: International Journal of Mental Health, Psychosocial Work and Counselling in Areas of Armed Conflict,* 2(2), 108–117.

———. (2005). Interventions for Survivors of the Tsunami Disaster: Report from Sri Lanka. *Journal of Traumatic Stress,* 18(3), 267–268.

———. (2008). Assessing Mental Health and Psychosocial Status in Communities Exposed to Traumatic Events: Sri Lanka as an Example. *American Journal of Orthopsychiatry,* 78(2), 229.

Ford, J. D., Campbell, K. A., Storzbach, D., Binder, L. M., Anger, W. K., & Rohlman, D. S. (2001). Posttraumatic Stress Symptomatology Is Associated with Unexplained Illness Attributed to Persian Gulf War Military Service. *Psychosomatic Medicine,* 63(5), 842–849.

Galappatti, A. (2003). What Is a Psychosocial Intervention? Mapping the Field in Sri Lanka. *Intervention,* 1(2), 3–17.

———. (2005). Psychosocial Work in the Aftermath of the Tsunami: Challenges for Service Provision in Batticaloa, Eastern Sri Lanka. *Intervention,* 1(1), 65–69.

Ganesan, M. (2006). Psychosocial Response to Disasters: Some Concerns. *International Review of Psychiatry,* 18(3), 241–247.

Gaughwin, P. (2008). Psychiatry's Problem Child: PTSD in the Forensic Context. Part 1. *Australasian Psychiatry: Bulletin of Royal Australian and New Zealand College of Psychiatrists,* 16(2), 104–108.

Ghodse, H., & Galea, S. (2006). Tsunami: Understanding Mental Health Consequences and the Unprecedented Response. *International Review of Psychiatry,* 18(3), 289–297.

Harold Merskey, D. M., & Piper, A. (2007). Posttraumatic Stress Disorder Is Overloaded. *Canadian Journal of Psychiatry,* 52(8), 499–500.

Heir, T., & Weisaeth, L. (2006). Back to Where It Happened: Self-Reported Symptom Improvement of Tsunami Survivors Who Returned to the Disaster Area. *Prehospital and Disaster Medicine: The Official Journal of the National Association of EMS Physicians and the World Association for Emergency and Disaster Medicine in Association with the Acute Care Foundation,* 21(2 Suppl. 2), 59–63.

Heir, T., & Weisaeth, L. (2008). Acute Disaster Exposure and Mental Health Complaints of Norwegian Tsunami Survivors Six Months Post Disaster. *Psychiatry,* 71(3), 266–276.

Hinton, D. E., Hinton, S. D., Loeum, R. J., Pich, V., & Pollack, M. H. (2008). The "Multiplex Model" of Somatic Symptoms: Application to Tinnitus among Traumatized Cambodian Refugees. *Transcultural Psychiatry,* 45(2), 287–317.

Hollifield, M., Hewage, C., Gunawardena, C. N., Kodituwakku, P., Bopagoda, K., & Weerarathnege, K. (2008). Symptoms and Coping in Sri Lanka 20–21 Months after the 2004 Tsunami. *British Journal of Psychiatry: The Journal of Mental Science,* 192(1), 39–44.

Jayasinghe, K. S. A., De Silva, D., Mendis, N., & Lie, R. K. (1998). Ethics of Resource Allocation in Developing Countries: The Case of Sri Lanka. *Social Science & Medicine,* 47(10), 1619–1625.

Johnson, H., & Thompson, A. (2008). The Development and Maintenance of Post-Traumatic Stress Disorder (PTSD) in Civilian Adult Survivors of War Trauma and Torture: A Review. *Clinical Psychology Review,* 28(1), 36–47.

Jones, E., Hodgins-Vermaas, R., McCartney, H., Everitt, B., Beech, C., Poynter, D., et al. (2002). Post-Combat Syndromes from the Boer War to the Gulf War: A Cluster Analysis of Their Nature and Attribution. *British Medical Journal,* 324(7333), 321.

Jones, E., Vermaas, R. H., McCartney, H., Beech, C., Palmer, I., Hyams, K., et al. (2003). Flashbacks and Post-Traumatic Stress Disorder: The Genesis of a 20th-Century Diagnosis. *British Journal of Psychiatry,* 182(2), 158–163.

Jones, E., Woolven, R., Durodie, B., & Wessely, S. (2004). Civilian Morale During the Second World War: Responses to Air Raids Re-examined. *Social History of Medicine,* 17(3), 463–479.

Jordan, K. (2006). A Case Study: How a Disaster Mental Health Volunteer Provided Spiritually, Culturally, and Historically Sensitive Trauma Training to Teacher-Counselors and Other Mental Health Professionals in Sri Lanka, 4 Weeks after the Tsunami. *Brief Treatment and Crisis Intervention,* 6(4), 316.

Kaplan, A. (2005, February). Tsunami Aftermath in Sri Lanka. *Psychiatric Times,* 22(2).

Keenan, P., & Royle, L. (2007). Vicarious Trauma and First Responders: A Case Study Utilizing Eye Movement Desensitization and Reprocessing (EMDR) as the Primary Treatment Modality. *International Journal of Emergency Mental Health,* 9(4), 291–298.

Kienzler, H. (2008). Debating War-Trauma and Post-Traumatic Stress Disorder (PTSD) in an Interdisciplinary Arena. *Social Science & Medicine,* 67(2), 218–227.

Kilshaw, S. (2008). Gulf War Syndrome: A Reaction to Psychiatry's Invasion of the Military? *Culture, Medicine and Psychiatry,* 32(2), 219–237.

Kinzie, J. D., & Goetz, R. R. (1996). A Century of Controversy Surrounding Posttraumatic Stress Stress-Spectrum Syndromes: The

Impact on *DSM-III* and *DSM-IV*. *Journal of Traumatic Stress,* 9(2), 159–179.

Kirmayer, L. J., Kienzler, H., Afana, A., & Pedersen, D. (in press). Trauma and Disasters in Social and Cultural Context. In D. Bhugra & C. Morgan, eds., *Principles of Social Psychiatry.* Wiley-Blackwell.

Kirmayer, L. J., Lemelson, R., & Barad, M. (2007). *Understanding Trauma: Integrating Biological, Clinical, and Cultural Perspectives.* Cambridge University Press.

Kleinman, A., & Becker, A. E. (1998). "Sociosomatics": The Contributions of Anthropology to Psychosomatic Medicine. *Journal of the American Psychosomatic Society* 60, 389–393.

Kumar, M. S., Murhekar, M. V., Hutin, Y., Subramanian, T., Ramachandran, V., & Gupte, M. D. (2007). Prevalence of Posttraumatic Stress Disorder in a Coastal Fishing Village in Tamil Nadu, India, after the December 2004 Tsunami. *American Journal of Public Health,* 97(1), 99–101.

Lange, G., Tiersky, L., DeLuca, J., Peckerman, A., Pollet, C., Policastro, T., et al. (1999). Psychiatric Diagnoses in Gulf War Veterans with Fatiguing Illness. *Psychiatry Research,* 89(1), 39–48.

Lau, J. T. F., Lau, M., Kim, J. H., & Tsui, H. Y. (2006). Impacts of Media Coverage on the Community Stress Level in Hong Kong after the Tsunami on 26 December 2004. *Journal of Epidemiology & Community Health,* 60(8), 675–682.

Lees-Haley, P. R., & Dunn, J. T. (1994). The Ability of Naive Subjects to Report Symptoms of Mild Brain Injury, Post-Traumatic Stress Disorder, Major Depression, and Generalized Anxiety Disorder. *Journal of Clinical Psychology,* 50(2), 252–256.

Leitch, M. L. (2007). Somatic Experiencing Treatment with Tsunami Survivors in Thailand: Broadening the Scope of Early Intervention. *Traumatology,* 13(3), 11.

Lilienfeld, S. O., Lynn, S. J., Kirsch, I., Chaves, J. F., Sarbin, T. R., Ganaway, G. K., et al. (1999). Dissociative Identity Disorder and the Sociocognitive Model: Recalling the Lessons of the Past. *Psychological Bulletin,* 125, 507–523.

Lutz, C. (1988). *Unnatural Emotions: Everyday Sentiments on a Micronesian Atoll and Their Challenge to Western Theory.* University of Chicago Press.

Lyn, T. E. (2005, January 3). Traumatised Tsunami Survivors to Take Years to Heal. *India News*.

Mahoney, J., Chandra, V., Gambheera, H., De Silva, T., & Suveendran, T. (2006). Responding to the Mental Health and Psychosocial Needs of the People of Sri Lanka in Disasters. *International Review of Psychiatry*, 18(6), 593–597.

Maier, T. (2006). Post-Traumatic Stress Disorder Revisited: Deconstructing the A-Criterion. *Medical Hypotheses*, 66(1), 103–106.

McHugh, P. R., & Treisman, G. (2007). PTSD: A Problematic Diagnostic Category. *Journal of Anxiety Disorders*, 21(2), 211–222.

McNally, R. J. (2004). Conceptual Problems with the *DSM-IV* Criteria for Posttraumatic Stress Disorder. In G. M. Rosen, ed., *Posttraumatic Stress Disorder: Issues and Controversies* (pp. 1–14).

Merridale, C. (2000). The Collective Mind: Trauma and Shell-Shock in Twentieth-Century Russia. *Journal of Contemporary History*, 35(1), 39.

Miller, G. (2005, August 12). The Tsunami's Psychological Aftermath. *Science*, 309.

Miller, K. E. (1999). Rethinking a Familiar Model: Psychotherapy and the Mental Health of Refugees. *Journal of Contemporary Psychotherapy*, 29(4), 283–306.

Miller, K. E., Kulkarni, M., & Kushner, H. (2006). Beyond Trauma-Focused Psychiatric Epidemiology: Bridging Research and Practice with War-Affected Populations. *American Journal of Orthopsychiatry*, 76(4), 409–422.

Miller, K. E., & Rasco, L. M. (2004). *The Mental Health of Refugees: Ecological Approaches to Healing and Adaptation*. Lawrence Erlbaum.

Neuner, F., Schauer, E., Catani, C., Ruf, M., & Elbert, T. (2006). Post-Tsunami Stress: A Study of Posttraumatic Stress Disorder in Children Living in Three Severely Affected Regions in Sri Lanka. *Journal of Traumatic Stress*, 19(3), 339–347.

Ng, B. Y. (2005). Grief revisited. *Annals of the Academy of Medicine Singapore*, 34(5), 352.

Nikapota, A. (2006). After the Tsunami: A Story from Sri Lanka. *International Review of Psychiatry*, 18(3), 275–279.

Norman, J. (2008, August 3). Mental Health Workers Becoming Standard in Disaster Relief Efforts. *Sunday Gazette-Mail* (Charleston, W. Va.).

Ofshe, R., Watters, E., (1996). *Making Monsters: False Memories, Psychotherapy, and Sexual Hysteria*. University of California Press.

Oyserman, D., Coon, H. M., & Kemmelmeier, M. (2002). Rethinking Individualism and Collectivism: Evaluation of Theoretical Assumptions and Meta-Analyses. *Psychological Bulletin*, 128(1), 3–72.

Page, D. (2005, December 1). New Study Demonstrates Long-Term Benefits of Psychotherapy for PTSD among Traumatized Adolescents. *UCLA News*.

Parker, C., Doctor, R. M., & Selvam, R. (2008). Somatic Therapy Treatment Effects with Tsunami Survivors. *Traumatology*, 14(3), 103.

Parker, T. (2006, May 5). Tsunami Prompts Women's Swimming Lessons. BBC News.

Pedersen, D. (2002). Political Violence, Ethnic Conflict, and Contemporary Wars: Broad Implications for Health and Social Well-Being. *Social Science & Medicine*, 55(2), 175–190.

Penn Psychologist to Provide Tsunami-Survivor Training. (2005, October 10). *Penn Medicine*.

Pityaratstian, N., Liamwanich, K., Ngamsamut, N., Narkpongphun, A., Chinajitphant, N., Burapakajornpong, N., et al. (2007). Cognitive-Behavioral Intervention for Young Tsunami Victims. *Journal of the Medical Association of Thailand*, 90(3), 518–523.

Piyavhatkul, N., Pairojkul, S., & Suphakunpinyo, C. (2008). Psychiatric Disorders in Tsunami-Affected Children in Ranong Province, Thailand. *Medical Principles and Practice*, 17(4), 290–295.

Pupavac, V. (2001a). Misanthropy without Borders: The International Children's Rights Regime. *Disasters*, 25(2), 95–112.

———. (2001b). Therapeutic Governance: Psycho-Social Intervention and Trauma Risk Management, *Disasters*, 25(4), 358–372.

———. (2004). Psychosocial Interventions and the Demoralization of Humanitarianism. *Journal of Biosocial Science*, 36(4), 491–504.

Raj, M. (2005, January 4). Psychological Therapy for Victims. *The Hindu* (India).

Rajkumar, A. P., Premkumar, T. S., & Tharyan, P. (2008). Coping with the Asian Tsunami: Perspectives from Tamil Nadu, India on the Determinants of Resilience in the Face of Adversity. *Social Science & Medicine*, 67(5), 844–853.

Regel, S. (2007). Post-Trauma Support in the Workplace: The Current Status and Practice of Critical Incident Stress Management and Psychological Debriefing within Organizations in the UK. *Occupational Medicine* (Oxford, England), 57(6), 411–416.

Richardson, N. (2006, May 15). UGA Doctoral Student Mahlet Endal Puts Her Counseling Preparation to Work for Victims of Tsunami in Sri Lanka. *Education Magazine* (U.S.).

Rose, S., Bisson, J., & Wessely, S. (2003). A Systematic Review of Single-Session Psychological Interventions ("Debriefing") Following Trauma. *Psychotherapy and Psychosomatics,* 72(4), 176–184.

Rose, S., Brewin, C. R., Andrews, B., & Kirk, M. (1999). A Randomized Controlled Trial of Individual Psychological Debriefing for Victims of Violent Crime. *Psychological Medicine,* 29(4), 793–799.

Rosen, G. (2004). *Posttraumatic Stress Disorder: Issues and Controversies.* Wiley.

Rosen, G. M., & Lilienfeld, S. O. (2008). Posttraumatic Stress Disorder: An Empirical Evaluation of Core Assumptions. *Clinical Psychology Review,* 28(5), 837–868.

Rosen, G. M., Spitzer, R. L., & McHugh, P. R. (2008). Problems with the Post-Traumatic Stress Disorder Diagnosis and Its Future in *DSM-V. British Journal of Psychiatry,* 192(1), 3.

Sajirawattakul, D. (2005, September 6). Blood Gathered for Tsunami-Trauma DNA Study. *The Nation.*

Schwartz, T., White, G. M., & Lutz, C. (1992). *New Directions in Psychological Anthropology.* Cambridge University Press.

Shah, S. A. (2006). Resistance to Cross-Cultural Psychosocial Efforts in Disaster and Trauma: Recommendations for Ethnomedical Competence. *Australasian Journal of Disaster and Trauma Studies,* 2006 (2).

Shatan, C. (1972). Post-Vietnam Syndrome. *New York Times,* 6.

Shell Shock. (1918). *California State Journal of Medicine,* 16(12), 515.

Shephard, B., & Cambridge, M. (2001). *A War of Nerves: Soldiers and Psychiatrists in the Twentieth Century.* American Psychiatric Association.

Silove, D., Steel, Z., & Psychol, M. (2006). Understanding Community Psychosocial Needs after Disasters: Implications for Mental Health Services. *Journal of Postgraduate Medicine,* 52(2), 121–125.

Silove, D., & Zwi, A. B. (2005). Translating Compassion into Psychosocial Aid after the Tsunami. *Lancet,* 365(9456), 269–271.

Sin, S. S., Chan, A., & Huak, C. Y. (2005). A Pilot Study of the Impact of the Asian Tsunami on a Group of Asian Media Workers. *International Journal of Emergency Mental Health,* 7(4), 299.

Solomon, Z., Bleich, A., Koslowsky, M., Kron, S., Lerer, B., & Waysman, M. (1991). Post-Traumatic Stress Disorder: Issues of Co-Morbidity. *Journal of Psychiatric Research,* 25(3), 89–94.

Somasundaram, D. (2007). Collective Trauma in Northern Sri Lanka: A Qualitative Psychosocial-Ecological Study. *International Journal of Mental Health Systems,* 1, 5.

Southwick, S. M., Morgan 3rd, C. A., Nicolaou, A. L., & Charney, D. S. (1997). Consistency of Memory for Combat-Related Traumatic Events in Veterans of Operation Desert Storm. *Journal of the American Psychiatric Association,* 154, 173–177.

Stevens, G., Byrne, S., Raphael, B., & Ollerton, R. (2008). Disaster Medical Assistance Teams: What Psychosocial Support Is Needed? *Prehospital and Disaster Medicine,* 23(2), 202.

Stone, R. (2005, December 9). In the Wake: Looking for Keys to Post-traumatic Stress. *Science,* 310.

Sumathipala, A. (n.d.). Written Submission to the Select Committee of Parliament to Recommend Steps to Minimize the Damages from Natural Disasters, http://www.forum4research.org/news/forum/written%20submission%20to%20the%20parliamentary%20select%20commitee%20fina.doc.

Sumathipala, A., & Siribaddana, S. (2005). Research and Clinical Ethics after the Tsunami: Sri Lanka. *Lancet,* 366(9495), 1418–1420.

Sumathipala, A., Siribaddana, S., Hewege, S., Lekamwattage, M., Athukorale, M., Siriwardhana, C., et al. (2008). Ethics Review Committee Approval and Informed Consent: An Analysis of Biomedical Publications Originating from Sri Lanka, *BMC Medical Ethics,* 9(1), 3.

Summerfield, D. (1999). A Critique of Seven Assumptions behind Psychological Trauma Programmes in War-Affected Areas. *Social Science & Medicine,* 48(10), 1449–1462.

———. (2001). The Invention of Post-Traumatic Stress Disorder and the Social Usefulness of a Psychiatric Category. *British Medical Journal,* 322, 95–98.

———. (2002). Effects of War: Moral Knowledge, Revenge, Reconciliation, and Medicalised Concepts of Recovery. *British Medical Journal,* 325, 1105–1107.

———. (2006). Survivors of the Tsunami: Dealing with Disaster. *Psychiatry,* 5(7), 255–256.

———. (2008). How Scientifically Valid Is the Knowledge Base of Global Mental Health? *British Medical Journal: Clinical Research Education*; 336(7651), 992–994.

Surface, D. (n.d.). Waves of Healing: Group Therapy with Tsunami Survivors. *Social Work Today,* 6(6), 30.

Thienkrua, W., Cardozo, B. L., Chakkraband, M. L., Guadamuz, T. E., Pengjuntr, W., Tantipiwatanaskul, P., et al. (2006). Symptoms of Posttraumatic Stress Disorder and Depression among Children in Tsunami-Affected Areas in Southern Thailand. *Journal of the American Medical Association,* 296(5), 549.

Trauma Risk for Tsunami Survivors. (2005, February 2). BBC News.

Tribe, R. (2007). Health Pluralism: A More Appropriate Alternative to Western Models of Therapy in the Context of the Civil Conflict and Natural Disaster in Sri Lanka? *Journal of Refugee Studies,* 20(1), 21.

Van Eenwyk, J. R. (2005, April 3). Relief Groups Can Create Unintended Chaos. *Seattle Post-Intelligencer.*

Van Hooff, M., McFarlane, A. C., Baur, J., Abraham, M., & Barnes, D. J. (2009). The Stressor Criterion-A1 and PTSD: A Matter of Opinion? *Journal of Anxiety Disorders,* 23(1), 77–86.

Van Ommeren, M., Saxena, S., & Saraceno, B. (2005). Mental and Social Health during and after Acute Emergencies: Emerging Consensus? *Bulletin of the World Health Organization,* 83, 71–75.

Ventevogel, P. (2008). From the Editor: The IASC Guidelines on Mental Health and Psychosocial Support in Emergency Settings, from Discussion to Implementation. *Intervention,* 6(3), 193.

Vijayakumar, L., Kannan, G. K., Kumar, B. G., & Devarajan, P. (2006). Do All Children Need Intervention after Exposure to Tsunami? *International Review of Psychiatry,* 18(6), 515–522.

von Peter, S. (2008). The Experience of "Mental Trauma" and its Transcultural Application. *Transcultural Psychiatry,* 45(4), 639–651.

Wentz, D. (2005). Shoring Up a Mental Health System. *Behavioral Health Management,* 25(5), 17–20.

Wessells, M., & Kostelny, K. (2005). *Assessing Afghan Children's Psychosocial Well-Being: A Multi-Modal Study of Intervention Outcomes.*

Christian Children's Fund, Oxford University, and Queen Margaret's University College.

Wickrama, K. A. S., & Kaspar, V. (2007). Family Context of Mental Health Risk in Tsunami-Exposed Adolescents: Findings from a Pilot Study in Sri Lanka. *Social Science & Medicine*, 64(3), 713–723.

Wickramage, K. (2006). Sri Lanka's Post-Tsunami Psychosocial Playground: Lessons for Future Psychosocial Programming and Interventions Following Disasters. *Intervention*, 4(2) 167–172.

Wilson, J. P., & Tang, C. S. (2007). *Cross-Cultural Assessment of Psychological Trauma and PTSD*. Springer.

Young, A. (1995a). *The Harmony of Illusions: Inventing Post-Traumatic Stress Disorder*. Princeton University Press.

———. (1995b). Reasons and Causes for Post-Traumatic Stress Disorder. *Transcultural Psychiatry*, 32(3), 287.

Yule, W. (2006). Theory, Training and Timing: Psychosocial Interventions in Complex Emergencies. *International Review of Psychiatry*, 18(3), 259–264.

Zarowsky, C. (2000). Trauma Stories: Violence, Emotion and Politics in Somali Ethiopia. *Transcultural Psychiatry*, 37(3), 383.

———. (2004). Writing Trauma: Emotion, Ethnography, and the Politics of Suffering among Somali Returnees in Ethiopia. *Culture, Medicine and Psychiatry*, 28(2), 189–209.

Chapter 3
The Shifting Mask of Schizophrenia in Zanzibar

It perhaps goes without saying that the work of Juli McGruder has been central to my thinking on schizophrenia. Her dissertation brought me to Zanzibar; her hospitality when I visited her was very gracious. A small group of researchers—Kim Hopper, Janis Hunter Jenkins, Robert John Barret, Byron Good, Sue Esteroff, Louis Sass, and Nancy Scheper-Hughes—formed the intellectual foundation on which McGruder built. All of these scholars, save the last, contributed to a remarkable book of papers entitled *Schizophrenia, Culture, and Subjectivity: The Edge of Experience*, which I highly recommend.

Other papers and resources I relied on include the following:

Allardyce, J., & Boydell, J. (2006). Environment and Schizophrenia. Review: The Wider Social Environment and Schizophrenia. *Schizophrenia Bulletin,* 32(4), 592.

Barrowclough, C., & Hooley, J. M. (2003). Attributions and Expressed Emotion: A Review. *Clinical Psychology Review,* 23(6), 849–880.

Birchwood, M., Mason, R., MacMillan, F., & Healy, J. (1993). Depression, Demoralization and Control over Psychotic Illness: A Comparison of Depressed and Non-Depressed Patients with a Chronic Psychosis. *Psychological Medicine,* 23(2), 387–395.

Breitborde, N. J. K., López, S. R., & Nuechterlein, K. H. (2009). Expressed Emotion, Human Agency, and Schizophrenia: Toward a New Model for the EE-Relapse Association. *Culture, Medicine and Psychiatry,* 33(1), 41–60.

Brekke, J. S., & Barrio, C. (1997). Cross-Ethnic Symptom Differences in Schizophrenia: The Influence of Culture and Minority Status. *Schizophrenia Bulletin,* 23(2), 305.

Brown, G. W., & Rutter, M. (1966). The Measurement of Family Activities and Relationships. *Human Relations,* 19, 241–263.

Butzlaff, R. L., & Hooley, J. M. (1998). Expressed Emotion and Psychiatric Relapse: A Meta-Analysis. *Archives of General Psychiatry,* 55, 547–552.

Cena, L., McGruder, J., & Tomlin, G. (2002). Representations of Race, Ethnicity, and Social Class in Case Examples. *American Journal of Occupational Therapy,* 56(2), 130–139.

Cochrane, R., & Bal, S. S. (1987). Migration and Schizophrenia: An Examination of Five Hypotheses. *Social Psychiatry and Psychiatric Epidemiology,* 22(4), 181–191.

Corrigan, P. W., & Watson, A. C. (2004). At Issue. Stop the Stigma: Call Mental Illness a Brain Disease. *Schizophrenia Bulletin,* 30(3), 477.

Craig, T. J., Siegel, C., Hopper, K., Lin, S., & Sartorius, N. (1997). Outcome in Schizophrenia and Related Disorders Compared between Developing and Developed Countries: A Recursive Partitioning Re-Analysis of the WHO DOSMD Data. *British Journal of Psychiatry,* 170(3), 229–233.

Davidson, L., & McGlashan, T. H. (1997). The Varied Outcomes of Schizophrenia. *Canadian Journal of Psychiatry,* 42, 34–43.

Dietrich, S., Beck, M., Bujantugs, B., Kenzine, D., Matschinger, H., &

Angermeyer, M. C. (2004). The Relationship between Public Causal Beliefs and Social Distance toward Mentally Ill People. *Australian and New Zealand Journal of Psychiatry,* 38(5), 348–354.

Earley, P. (2006). *Crazy: A Father's Search through America's Mental Health Madness.* Putnam.

Estroff, S. E., Penn, D. L., & Toporek, J. R. (2004). From Stigma to Discrimination: An Analysis of Community Efforts to Reduce the Negative Consequences of Having a Psychiatric Disorder and Label. *Schizophrenia Bulletin,* 30(3), 493.

Fàbrega Jr., H. (2001). Culture and History in Psychiatric Diagnosis and Practice. *Psychiatric Clinics of North America,* 24(3), 391–405.

Fàbrega Jr., H. (1991). The Culture and History of Psychiatric Stigma in Early Modern and Modern Western Societies: A Review of Recent Literature. *Comprehensive Psychiatry,* 32(2), 97.

Fincher, C. L., Thornhill, R., Murray, D. R., & Schaller, M. (2008). Pathogen Prevalence Predicts Human Cross-Cultural Variability in Individualism/Collectivism. Proceedings. *Biological Sciences/The Royal Society,* 275(1640), 1279–1285.

Fisher, J. D., & Farina, A. (1979). Consequences of Beliefs about the Nature of Mental Disorders. *Journal of Abnormal Psychology,* 88(3), 320–327.

Good, B. (1994). *Medicine, Rationality, and Experience: An Anthropological Perspective.* Cambridge University Press.

Granger, D. A. (1994). Recovery from Mental Illness: A First-Person Perspective of an Emerging Paradigm. In Ohio Department of Mental Health, *Recovery: The New Force in Mental Health* (pp. 1–13). Author.

Halliburton, M. (2005). "Just Some Spirits": The Erosion of Spirit Possession and the Rise of "Tension" in South India. *Medical Anthropology,* 24(2), 111–144.

Hashemi, A. H., & Cochrane, R. (1999). Expressed Emotion and Schizophrenia: A Review of Studies across Cultures. *International Review of Psychiatry,* 11(2), 219–224.

Hooley, J. M. (1998). Expressed Emotion and Locus of Control. *Journal of Nervous and Mental Disease,* 186(6), 374–378.

———. (2007). Expressed Emotion and Relapse of Psychopathology. *Annual Review of Clinical Psychology,* 3: 329–352.

Hopper, K., Harrison, G., Janca, A., & Sartorius, N. (2007). *Recovery from Schizophrenia: An International Perspective. A Report from the WHO Collaborative Project, the International Study of Schizophrenia.* Oxford University Press.

Hopper, K., & Wanderling, J. (2000). Revisiting the Developed versus Developing Country Distinction in Course and Outcome in Schizophrenia: Results from Isos, the WHO Collaborative Followup Project. *Schizophrenia Bulletin,* 26(4), 835.

Jablensky, A. (1987). Multicultural Studies and the Nature of Schizophrenia: A Review. *Journal of the Royal Society of Medicine,* 80(3), 162.

————. (1995). Schizophrenia: Recent Epidemiologic Issues. *Epidemiologic Reviews,* 17(1), 10–20.

————. (1997). The 100-Year Epidemiology of Schizophrenia. *Schizophrenia Research,* 28(2–3), 111–125.

————. (2006). The Epidemiology of Schizophrenia. *Australian and New Zealand Journal of Psychiatry,* 40(5), 503.

Jenkins, J. H. (1997). Subjective Experience of Persistent Schizophrenia and Depression among U.S. Latinos and Euro-Americans. *British Journal of Psychiatry,* 171(1), 20–25.

————. (1998a). Conceptions of Schizophrenia as a Problem of Nerves: A Cross-Cultural Comparison of Mexican-Americans and Anglo-Americans. *Social Science & Medicine,* 26(12), 1233.

————. (1988b). Ethnopsychiatric Interpretations of Schizophrenic Illness: The Problem of Nervios within Mexican-American Families. *Culture, Medicine and Psychiatry,* 12(3), 301–329.

————. (1991). Anthropology, Expressed Emotion, and Schizophrenia. *Ethos,* 19(4), 387–431.

————. (1992). Too Close for Comfort: Schizophrenia and Emotional Overinvolvement among Mexicano Families. In A. Gaines, ed., *Ethnopsychiatry: The Cultural Construction of Professional and Folk Psychiatries* (pp. 203–221). State University of New York Press.

Jenkins, J. H., & Barrett, R. J. (2003). *Schizophrenia, Culture, and Subjectivity.* Cambridge University Press.

Jenkins, J. H., & Karno, M. (1992). The Meaning of Expressed Emotion: Theoretical Issues Raised by Cross-Cultural Research. *American Journal of Psychiatry,* 149, 9–21.

Jenkins, J. H., & Schumacher, J. G. (1999). Family Burden of Schizophrenia and Depressive Illness: Specifying the Effects of Ethnicity, Gender and Social Ecology. *British Journal of Psychiatry,* 174(1), 31–38.

Jilek, W. G. (1998). Transcultural Psychiatry, Quo Vadis. *Transcultural Psychology Newsletter,* 16(1), 1–10.

Kent, H., & Read, J. (1998). Measuring Consumer Participation in Mental Health Services: Are Attitudes Related to Professional Orientation? *International Journal of Social Psychiatry,* 44(4), 295–310.

Kleinman, A. (1987). Anthropology and Psychiatry. The Role of Culture in Cross-Cultural Research on Illness. *British Journal of Psychiatry,* 151(4), 447–454.

———. (1988). *The Illness Narratives: Suffering, Healing, and the Human Condition.* Basic Books.

Kleinman, A., & Cohen, A. (1997). Psychiatry's Global Challenge. *Scientific American,* 276(3), 86–89.

Kopelowicz, A., Zarate, R., Gonzalez, V., Lopez, S. R., Ortega, P., Obregon, N., et al. (2002). Evaluation of Expressed Emotion in Schizophrenia: A Comparison of Caucasians and Mexican-Americans. *Schizophrenia Research,* 55(1–2), 179–186.

Kulhara, P. (1994). Outcome of Schizophrenia: Some Transcultural Observations with Particular Reference to Developing Countries. *European Archives of Psychiatry and Clinical Neuroscience,* 244(5), 227–235.

Kymalainen, J. A., de Mamani, A. G., & Amy, G. (2008). Expressed Emotion, Communication Deviance, and Culture in Families of Patients with Schizophrenia: A Review of the Literature. *Cultural Diversity and Ethnic Minority Psychology,* 14(2), 85.

Langer, E. J., & Abelson, R. P. (1974). A Patient by Any Other Name: Clinician Group Difference in Labeling Bias. *Journal of Consulting and Clinical Psychology,* 42(1), 4–9.

Leff, J., Wig, N. N., Ghosh, A., Bedi, H., Menon, D. K., Kuipers, L., et al. (1987). Expressed Emotion and Schizophrenia in North India: Influence of Relatives' Expressed Emotion on the Course of Schizophrenia in Chandigarh. *British Journal of Psychiatry,* 151(2), 166–173.

Lefley, H. P. (1990). Culture and Chronic Mental Illness. *Hospital & Community Psychiatry,* 41(3), 277–286.

Lutz, C. (1988). *Unnatural Emotions: Everyday Sentiments on a Micronesian Atoll and their Challenge to Western Theory.* University of Chicago Press.

Marom, S., Munitz, H., Jones, P. B., Weizman, A., & Hermesh, H. (2002). Familial Expressed Emotion: Outcome and Course of Israeli Patients with Schizophrenia. *Schizophrenia Bulletin,* 28(4), 731.

McGrath, J. J. (2005). Myths and Plain Truths about Schizophrenia Epidemiology: The Nape Lecture 2004. *Acta Psychiatrica Scandinavica,* 111(1), 4–11.

———. (2006). Variations in the Incidence of Schizophrenia: Data versus Dogma. *Schizophrenia Bulletin,* 32(1), 195–197.

———. (2007). The Surprisingly Rich Contours of Schizophrenia Epidemiology. *Archives of General Psychiatry,* 64(1), 14.

McGruder, J. (1999). Madness in Zanzibar: "Schizophrenia" in Three Families in the "Developing" World. Ph.D. dissertation, University of Washington.

———. (2002). Life Experience Is Not a Disease, or Why Medicalizing Madness Is Counterproductive to Recovery. In C. Brown, ed., *Recovery and Wellness: Models of Hope and Empowerment for People with Mental Illness* (pp. 59–80), Routledge.

Mehta, S., & Farina, A. (1997). Is Being Sick Really Better? Effect of the Disease View of Mental Disorder on Stigma. *Journal of Social and Clinical Psychology,* 16(4), 405–419.

Mezzich, J. E., Kirmayer, L. J., Kleinman, A., Fabrega Jr., H., et al. (1999). The Place of Culture in *DSM-IV. Journal of Nervous & Mental Disease,* 187(8), 457.

Neugeboren, J. (2003). *Imagining Robert* (p. 313). Rutgers University Press.

Oyserman, D., Coon, H. M., & Kemmelmeier, M. (2002). Rethinking Individualism and Collectivism: Evaluation of Theoretical Assumptions and Meta-Analyses. *Psychological Bulletin,* 128(1), 3–72.

Oyserman, D., & Lee, S. W. (2008). Does Culture Influence What and How We Think? Effects of Priming Individualism and Collectivism. *Psychological Bulletin,* 134(2), 311.

Prince, R. H. (1992). Religious Experience and Psychopathology: Cross-Cultural. *Religion and Mental Health,* 281.

Prince, R. H., & Reiss, M. (1990). Psychiatry and the Irrational: Does Our Scientific World View Interfere with the Adaptation of Psychotics? *Psychiatric Journal of the University of Ottawa: Revue de psychiatrie de l'Université d'Ottawa,* 15(3), 137.

Read, J., Haslam, N., Sayce, L., & Davies, E. (2006). Prejudice and Schizophrenia: A Review of the "Mental Illness Is an Illness Like Any Other" Approach. *Acta Psychiatrica Scandinavica,* 114(5), 303–318.

Sartorius, N., Gulbinat, W., Harrison, G., Laska, E., & Siegel, C. (1996). Long-Term Follow-Up of Schizophrenia in 16 Countries. *Social Psychiatry and Psychiatric Epidemiology,* 31(5), 249–258.

Sass, L. A. (1994). Civilized Madness: Schizophrenia, Self-Consciousness and the Modern Mind. *History of the Human Sciences,* 7, 83–120.

Scheper-Hughes, N. (1985). Culture, Scarcity, and Maternal Thinking: Maternal Detachment and Infant Survival in a Brazilian Shantytown. *Ethos,* 291–317.

———. (1993). *Death without Weeping: The Violence of Everyday Life in Brazil.* University of California Press.

———. (2001). *Saints, Scholars, and Schizophrenics: Mental Illness in Rural Ireland.* University of California Press.

Schnittker, J. (2008). An Uncertain Revolution: Why the Rise of a Genetic Model of Mental Illness Has Not Increased Tolerance. *Social Science & Medicine,* 67(9), 1370–1381.

Stompe, T., Friedman, A., Ortwein, G., Strobl, R., Chaudhry, H. R., Najam, N., et al. (1999). Comparison of Delusions among Schizophrenics in Austria and in Pakistan. *Psychopathology,* 32, 225–234.

Stompe, T., Karakula, H., Rudaleviciene, P., Okribelashvili, N., Chaudhry, H. R., Idemudia, E. E., et al. (2006). The Pathoplastic Effect of Culture on Psychotic Symptoms in Schizophrenia. *World Cultural Psychiatry Research Review,* 1(3/4), 157–163.

Stout, P. A., Villegas, J., & Jennings, N. A. (2004). Images of Mental Illness in the Media: Identifying Gaps in the Research. *Schizophrenia Bulletin,* 30(3), 543.

Suhail, K., & Cochrane, R. (2002). Effect of Culture and Environment on the Phenomenology of Delusions and Hallucinations. *International Journal of Social Psychiatry,* 48(2), 126.

Swift, C. R. (2002). *Dar Days* (p. 211). University Press of America.

Torrey, E. F. (1988). *Surviving Schizophrenia: A Family Manual.* Harper Perennial.

Weisman, A. G. (1997). Understanding Cross-Cultural Prognostic Variability for Schizophrenia. *Cultural Diversity and Mental Health,* 3(1), 23.

Wig, N. N., Bedi, D. K., Leff, J., Kuipers, L., Ghosh, A., Day, R., et al. (1987). Distribution of Expressed Emotion Components among Relatives of Schizophrenic Patients in Aarhus and Chandigarh. *British Journal of Psychiatry,* 151, 160–165.

Chapter 4

The Mega-Marketing of Depression in Japan

The scholars at McGill University are overrepresented in this book because that university is a hotbed for the study of cross-cultural psychiatry. That fact, I believe, has much to do with Laurence Kirmayer, whose work and leadership in the field informs not just this chapter but this entire book. Junko Kitanaka, Kirmayer's former graduate student, was as generous as her mentor with her time and guidance. The history of the evolution of Japanese understanding of depression relies critically on her dissertation—in particular, the recounting of the suicide of Oshima Ichiro and the public attention surrounding suicide from overwork. Her book on the history of depression in Japan will be out within a year or two, and I will be first in line at the bookstore to snap it up. David Healy was an inspiration both for his research on the science behind SSRIs and for his dogged courage.

Other resources include the following:

Ailing Crown Princess Steadily Improving. (2008, December 24). *Japan Times.*

Angell, M. (2009, January 15). Drug Companies and Doctors: A Story of Corruption. *New York Review of Books.*

Applbaum, K. (2004a). *The Marketing Era: From Professional Practice to Global Provisioning.* Routledge.

———. (2004b). How to Organize a Psychiatric Congress. *Anthropological Quarterly,* 77(2), 303–310.

———. (2006). Pharmaceutical Marketing and the Invention of the Medical Consumer. *PLoS Medicine,* 3(4), 445.

Ballenger, J. C., Davidson, J. R., Lecrubier, Y., Nutt, D. J., et al. (2001). A Proposed Algorithm for Improved Recognition and Treatment of the Depression/Anxiety Spectrum in Primary Care. *Primary Care Companion to the Journal of Clinical Psychiatry,* 3(2), 44.

Ballenger, J. C., Davidson, J. R., Lecrubier, Y., Nutt, D. J., Kirmayer, L. J., Lepine, J. P., et al. (2001). Consensus Statement on Transcultural Issues in Depression and Anxiety from the International Consensus Group on Depression and Anxiety. *Journal of Clinical Psychiatry,* 62(13), 47–55.

Barbui, C., Esposito, E., & Cipriani, A. (2009). Selective Serotonin Reuptake Inhibitors and Risk of Suicide: A Systematic Review of Observational Studies. *Canadian Medical Association Journal,* 180(3), 291.

Berger, D., & Fukunishi, I. (1996). Psychiatric Drug Development in Japan. *Science,* 273(5273), 318.

Bhugra, D., & Mastrogianni, A. (2004). Globalisation and Mental Disorders Overview with Relation to Depression. *British Journal of Psychiatry,* 184(1), 10–20.

Breslau, J. (2000). Globalizing Disaster Trauma: Psychiatry, Science, and Culture after the Kobe Earthquake. *Ethos,* 28(2), 174–197.

Calabrese, J. R., Kasper, S., Johnson, G., Tajima, O., Vieta, E., Yatham, L. N., et al. (2004). International Consensus Group on Bipolar I Depression Treatment Guidelines. *Journal of Clinical Psychiatry,* 65(4), 571.

Carta, M. G., Coppo, P., Reda, M. A., Hardoy, M. C., & Carpiniello, B. (n.d.). Depression and Social Change: From Transcultural Psychiatry to a Constructivist Model. *Epidemiologia e psichiatria sociale,* 10(1), 46.

Chan, A. W. (2008). Bias, Spin, and Misreporting: Time for Full Access to Trial Protocols and Results. *PLoS Medicine,* 5(11), e230.

Chen, H., Guarnaccia, P. J., & Chung, H. (2003). Self-Attention as a Mediator of Cultural Influences on Depression. *International Journal of Social Psychiatry,* 49(3), 192.

Currie, J. (2005). The Marketization of Depression: The Prescribing of SSRI Antidepressants to Women. *Women and Health Protection,* 1–27.

Ghaemi, N. (2008, December 7). Data, Dollars, and Drugs, Part I: The Ethics of Medicine. *Psychology Today.* Retrieved July 23, 2009.

Grassley, C. (2008, June 4). Payments to Physicians. *Congressional Record.*

Groleau, D., Young, A., & Kirmayer, L. J. (2006). The McGill Illness Narrative Interview (MINI): An Interview Schedule to Elicit Meanings and Modes of Reasoning Related to Illness Experience. *Transcultural Psychiatry,* 43(4), 671.

Gruenberg, A. M., Goldstein, R. D., & Pincus, H. A. (2005). Classification of Depression: Research and Diagnostic Criteria: *DSM-IV* and *ICD-10*. In *Biology of Depression: From Novel Insights to Therapeutic Strategies.* Wiley-VCH.

Gunnell, D., & Ashby, D. (2004). Antidepressants and Suicide: What Is the Balance of Benefit and Harm (Vol. 329, pp. 34–38). BMJ Publishing Group.

Gunnell, D., Saperia, J., & Ashby, D. (2005). Selective Serotonin Reuptake Inhibitors (SSRIS) and Suicide in Adults: Meta-Analysis of Drug Company Data from Placebo Controlled, Randomised Controlled Trials Submitted to the MHRA's Safety Review. *British Medical Journal,* 330(7488), 385.

Healy, D. (1997). *The Antidepressant Era.* Harvard University Press.

———. (2002). *The Creation of Psychopharmacology.* Harvard University Press.

———. (2004a). *Let Them Eat Prozac: The Unhealthy Relationship between the Pharmaceutical Industry and Depression.* New York University Press.

———. (2004b). Shaping the Intimate: Influences on the Experience of Everyday Nerves. *Social Studies of Science,* 34(2), 219.

———. (2008). *Psychiatric Drugs Explained.* Churchill Livingstone.

Healy, D., & Whitaker, C. (2003). Antidepressants and Suicide: Risk-Benefit Conundrums. *Journal of Psychiatry and Neuroscience,* 28(5), 331–339.

Horwitz, A. V., & Wakefield, J. C. (2007). *The Loss of Sadness: How Psychiatry Transformed Normal Sorrow into Depressive Disorder.* Oxford University Press.

Keller, M. B., Ryan, N. D., Strober, M., Klein, R. G., Kutcher, S. P., Birmaher, B., et al. (2001). Efficacy of Paroxetine in the Treatment of Adolescent Major Depression: A Randomized, Controlled Trial. *Journal of the American Academy of Child and Adolescent Psychiatry,* 40(7), 762.

Kirmayer, L. J. (1989). Cultural Variations in the Response to Psychiatric Disorders and Emotional Distress. *Social Science & Medicine,* 29(3), 327.

———. (1999). Rhetorics of the Body: Medically Unexplained Symptoms in Sociocultural Perspective. In *Somatoform Disorders: A Worldwide Perspective* (pp. 271–286). Springer-Verlag Telos.

———. (2001). Cultural Variations in the Clinical Presentation of

Depression and Anxiety: Implications for Diagnosis and Treatment. *Journal of Clinical Psychiatry,* 62, 22–30.

———. (2002). Psychopharmacology in a Globalizing World: The Use of Antidepressants in Japan. *Transcultural Psychiatry,* 39(3), 295.

———. (2005). Culture, Context and Experience in Psychiatric Diagnosis. *Psychopathology,* 38(4), 192–196.

———. (2006a). Beyond the "New Cross-Cultural Psychiatry": Cultural Biology, Discursive Psychology and the Ironies of Globalization. *Transcultural Psychiatry,* 43(1), 126.

———. (2006b). Culture and Psychotherapy in a Creolizing World. *Transcultural Psychiatry,* 43(2), 163.

———. (2007). Psychotherapy and the Cultural Concept of the Person. *Transcultural Psychiatry,* 44(2), 232.

Kirmayer, L. J., & Groleau, D. (2001). Affective Disorders in Cultural Context. *Psychiatric Clinics of North America,* 24(3), 465–478.

Kirmayer, L. J., & Looper, K. J. (2006). Abnormal Illness Behaviour: Physiological, Psychological and Social Dimensions of Coping with Distress. *Current Opinion in Psychiatry,* 19(1), 54.

Kirmayer, L. J., & Sartorius, N. (2007). Cultural Models and Somatic Syndromes. *Psychosomatic Medicine,* 69(9), 832.

Kirmayer, L. J., & Young, A. (1998). Culture and Somatization: Clinical, Epidemiological, and Ethnographic Perspectives. *Psychosomatic Medicine,* 60, 420–430.

Kitanaka, J. (2006). Society in Distress: The Psychiatric Production of Depression in Contemporary Japan. PhD dissertation, Department of Anthropology, McGill University.

———. (2008). Diagnosing Suicides of Resolve: Psychiatric Practice in Contemporary Japan. *Culture, Medicine and Psychiatry,* 32(2), 152–176.

Kleinman, A. (2001). A Psychiatric Perspective on Global Change. *Harvard Review of Psychiatry,* 9(1), 46–47.

——— (2004). Culture and Depression. *New England Journal of Medicine,* 351, 951–953.

Kleinman, A., Lakoff, A., & Petryna, A. (2007). *Global Pharmaceuticals.* Duke University Press.

Lacasse, J. R., & Leo, J. (2005). Serotonin and Depression: A Disconnect between the Advertisements and the Scientific Literature. *PLoS Medicine,* 2(12), 1211.

Lakoff, A. (2004). The Anxieties of Globalization:: Antidepressant Sales and Economic Crisis in Argentina. *Social Studies of Science,* 34(2), 247.

———. (2007). The Right Patients for the Drug: Managing the Placebo Effect in Antidepressant Trials. *BioSocieties,* 2(01), 57–71.

Landers, P. (2002, October 9). Drug Companies Push Japan to Change View of Depression. *Wall Street Journal.*

Lee, S. (1999). Diagnosis Postponed: Shenjing Shuairuo and the Transformation of Psychiatry in Post-Mao China. *Culture, Medicine and Psychiatry,* 23(3), 349–380.

Lepine, J. P. (2001). Epidemiology, Burden, and Disability in Depression and Anxiety. *Journal of Clinical Psychiatry,* 62, 4–12.

Lock, M. (1995). *Encounters with Aging: Mythologies of Menopause in Japan and North America.* University of California Press.

McHenry, L. (2006). Ethical Issues in Psychopharmacology. *British Medical Journal,* 32(7), 405.

Mezzich, J. E., Kirmayer, L. J., Kleinman, A., Fàbrega Jr., H., Parron, D. L., Good, B. J., et al. (1999). The Place of Culture in *DSM-IV. Journal of Nervous and Mental Disease,* 187(8), 457.

Moynihan, R., Doran, E., & Henry, D. (2008). Disease Mongering Is Now Part of the Global Health Debate. *PLoS Medicine,* 5(5), e106.

Olfson, M., & Marcus, S. C. (2008). A Case-Control Study of Antidepressants and Attempted Suicide during Early Phase Treatment of Major Depressive Episodes. *Journal of Clinical Psychiatry,* 69(3), 425–432.

Ozawa-de Silva, C. (2008). Too Lonely to Die Alone: Internet Suicide Pacts and Existential Suffering in Japan. *Culture, Medicine and Psychiatry,* 32(4), 516–551.

Petryna, A., Lakoff, A., & Kleinman, A. (2006). *Global Pharmaceuticals: Ethics, Markets, Practices.* Duke University Press.

Read, J., Haslam, N., Sayce, L., & Davies, E. (2006). Prejudice and Schizophrenia: A Review of the "Mental Illness Is an Illness Like Any Other" Approach. *Acta Psychiatrica Scandinavica,* 114(5), 303–318.

Rihmer, Z., & Akiskal, H. (2006). Do Antidepressants T(h)reat(en) Depressives? Toward a Clinically Judicious Formulation of the Antidepressant-Suicidality FDA Advisory in Light of Declining National Suicide Statistics from Many Countries. *Journal of Affective Disorders,* 94(1–3), 3–13.

Schulz, K. (2004, August 22). Did Antidepressants Depress Japan? *New York Times Magazine.*

Stotland, N. (2009, February 26). Drug Companies and Doctors: An Exchange. *New York Review of Books.*

Summerfield, D. (2006). Depression: Epidemic or Pseudo-Epidemic? *Journal of the Royal Society of Medicine, 99,* 161–162.

Tajima, O., et al. (2001). Mental Health Care in Japan: Recognition and Treatment of Depression and Anxiety Disorders. *Journal of Clinical Psychiatry,* Suppl., 62(13), 39–46.

Tanaka-Matsumi, J., & Marsella, A. J. (1976). Cross-Cultural Variations in the Phenomenological Experience of Depression: I. Word Association Studies. *Journal of Cross-Cultural Psychology, 7*(4), 379.

Teicher, M. H., Glod, C. A., & Cole, J. O. (1990). Emergence of Intense Suicidal Preoccupation during Fluoxetine Treatment. *American Journal of Psychiatry. 147,* 207–210.

Teicher, M. H., Glod, C. A., & Cole, J. O. (1993). Antidepressant Drugs and the Emergence of Suicidal Tendencies. *Drug Safety, 8*(3), 186.

Thomas, P., Bracken, P., Cutler, P., Hayward, R., May, R., & Yasmeen, S. (2005). Challenging the Globalisation of Biomedical Psychiatry. *Journal of Public Mental Health, 4*(3), 23–32.

Tsurumi, W. (1993). *The Complete Manual of Suicide.* Ohta Shuppan.

Valenstein, E. S., & Berger, L. S. (2001). Blaming the Brain: The Truth about Drugs and Mental Health. *Psychoanalytic Psychology, 18*(1), 184–187.

Ware, N. C., & Kleinman, A. (1992). Culture and Somatic Experience: The Social Course of Illness in Neurasthenia and Chronic Fatigue Syndrome. *Psychosomatic Medicine,* 546–560.

Weissman, M. M. (1998). The Antidepressant Era. *New England Journal of Medicine, 338,* 1475–1476.

Whittington, C. J., Kendall, T., Fonagy, P., Cottrell, D., Cotgrove, A., & Boddington, E. (2004). Selective Serotonin Reuptake Inhibitors in Childhood Depression: Systematic Review of Published versus Unpublished Data. *Lancet, 363*(9418), 1341–1345.

Yudofsky, H. R. (Ed.). (2003). *The American Psychiatric Press Textbook of Clinical Psychiatry* (Vol. 4). American Psychiatric Publishing.

Conclusion

Belluck, P. (2009, April 8). Recession Anxiety Seeps into Everyday Lives. *New York Times.*

Chisholm, D., Flisher, A. J., Lund, C., Patel, V., Saxena, S., Thornicroft, G., et al. (2007). Scale Up Services for Mental Disorders: A Call for Action. *Lancet,* 370(9594), 1241–1252.

More Than 300 New Medicines Being Developed for Mental Illnesses. (n.d.). PhRMA: New Medicine, New Hope. Retrieved from http://www.phrma.org/news_room/press_releases/more_than_300_new_medicines_being_developed_for_mental_illness/.

Seligman, R., & Kirmayer, L. J. (2008). Dissociative Experience and Cultural Neuroscience: Narrative, Metaphor and Mechanism. *Culture, Medicine and Psychiatry,* 32(1), 31–64.

Stier, K. (2009, February 9). Suicides: Watching for Recession Spike. *Time.*

Acknowledgments

I had several insightful readers at critical stages of this project. Po Bronson, Charis Conn, Rob Riddell, and my wife, Rebecca Watters, assisted me with everything from word choice to finding my way out of the conceptual labyrinths that these long chapters sometimes created. Others read portions as needed, including Alan Burdick, Laura Fraser, Michal Story, Todd Oppenheimer, and Eleanor Wendell. I'm indebted to my agent, Chris Calhoun, a champion for this project from the very beginning. At Free Press I've been pleased to work with Dominick Anfuso, who gave this book his thoughtful attention during a challenging year. Leah Miller was critically important in the creation of this book. My thanks also go to copyeditor Judith Hoover. Michal Story transcribed many of the interviews and gave me moral support as well. Kasie Cheung provided Chinese translation. Joelle Jaffe worked as my researcher on the anorexia and schizophrenia chapters and helped me think through the approach for the rest of the book. Encouragement from my mother, Mary Pulliam Watters, and my brother, Aaron Watters, was essential. This book was written at the San Francisco Writers' Grotto.

Index

About the Author

Ethan Watters is the author of *Urban Tribes,* an examination of the mores of the "never-marrieds," and the coauthor of *Making Monsters,* a groundbreaking indictment of the recovered memory movement. A frequent contributor to *The New York Times Magazine, Discover, Men's Journal, Wired,* and This American Life, he lives in San Francisco with his wife and children.